'Vanessa May's courageous survival of devastating personal bereavement combines with extensive professional experience to make this a deeply insightful guide into working sensitively and confidently with clients affected by trauma and the complexity of loss or unprocessed grief. I believe this is the essential "go to" handbook for every therapist, wellness coach or health professional. This is now required reading for our wellbeing coaching students.'

Elaine Wilkins, founder of Chrysalis Effect Health and author of The Trauma Informed Wellbeing Coaching Accreditation for Health Professionals

'I would highly recommend Vanessa May's book to any nutritional therapist, or indeed any health professional, to give them an understanding of the devastating impact that grief can have on an individual's health. If you are working with a client who is stricken with grief, unless their emotional needs are heard and supported, you may well find that they don't respond to your advice as you might hope or expect and that their grief dramatically hinders any improvements in their health – mental and physical – despite your best efforts. This book gives invaluable advice and insight on how to work sympathetically with grieving clients in order to support their individual health needs, both mental and physical.'

Kate Alexander, BANT-registered nutritionist, BANT membership manager

'Grief is messy and there's a lot of it about. Grief can contribute to chronic disease – even kill, yet most practitioners are unaware of its consequences. Vanessa May ably details the key nutritional support for grieving clients, while providing an excellent blueprint for understanding grief's impact on the gut and nervous system. A well-written, "easy" read, despite its subject, and a vital missing link in practitioner education.'

Simon Martin, editor of IHCAN *magazine*

Supporting Your
Grieving Client

of related interest

Integrative Wellness Coaching
A Handbook for Therapists and Counsellors
Laurel Alexander
ISBN 978 1 83997 089 4
eISBN 978 1 83997 090 0

Case Studies in Personalized Nutrition
Edited by Angela Walker
ISBN 978 8 4819 394 9
eISBN 978 0 85701 351 4

The Functional Nutrition Cookbook
Addressing Biochemical Imbalances through Diet
Lorraine Nicolle and Christine Bailey
ISBN 978 1 84819 079 5
eISBN 978 0 85701 052 0

Supporting Your
GRIEVING CLIENT

A GUIDE FOR WELLNESS PRACTITIONERS

Vanessa May

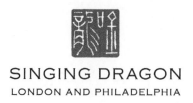

SINGING DRAGON
LONDON AND PHILADELPHIA

First published in Great Britain in 2023 by Singing Dragon,
an imprint of Jessica Kingsley Publishers
An imprint of Hodder & Stoughton Ltd
An Hachette Company

1

Copyright © Vanessa May 2023

The right of Vanessa May to be identified as the Author of the Work has been asserted by her in accordance with the Copyright, Designs and Patents Act 1988.

Quotes on pages 41, 72 and 190 are reproduced from May, 2022 with kind permission from John Hunt Publishing Ltd.

Front cover image source: Shutterstock®. The cover image is for illustrative purposes only, and any person featuring is a model.

A CIP catalogue record for this title is available from the British Library and the Library of Congress

ISBN 978 1 83997 347 5
eISBN 978 1 83997 348 2

Printed and bound by CPI Group (UK) Ltd, Croydon CR0 4YY

Jessica Kingsley Publishers' policy is to use papers that are natural, renewable and recyclable products and made from wood grown in sustainable forests. The logging and manufacturing processes are expected to conform to the environmental regulations of the country of origin.

Jessica Kingsley Publishers
Carmelite House
50 Victoria Embankment
London EC4Y 0DZ

www.singingdragon.com

Contents

Acknowledgements

With thanks to all at Singing Dragon: to Carys Homer, Masooma Malik and especially Claire Wilson, whose idea it was to write this book on how wellness practitioners might support a bereaved client. It wasn't until I started my research for the book that I realized just how much there might be a need for it.

Thank you to Tom Sandford for taking my simplistic sketches and illegible handwriting and turning them into illustrations that visually enhance the book.

With thanks to my lovely and very courageous daughter and to my mum, for her unconditional love and support. They both walk with me on this very challenging path of grieving multiple traumatic losses.

With the utmost heartfelt thanks to my husband. Before he died, he read my early work on this book. He unfailingly supported and encouraged my writing, on this and my first book *Love Untethered: How to Live When Your Child Dies*, understanding that writing was my way of processing the death of our beloved son.

This book is dedicated to him and to my beautiful boy, two shining souls who now guide me from a different dimension not too far away. My bond with them continues; our love unending.

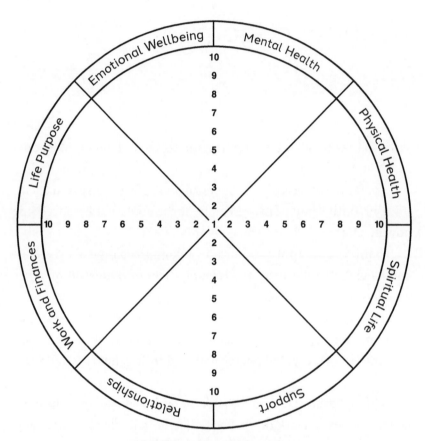

THE HOLISTIC GRIEF WHEEL.
A VISUAL TOOL FOR WELLNESS PRACTITIONERS TO USE
WITH THEIR CLIENTS IN ORDER TO IDENTIFY THE AREAS
MOST AFFECTED BY GRIEF (SEE CHAPTER 10).

Introduction

Supporting Your Grieving Client is for you if you're a wellness practitioner or alternative therapist who is likely, at some point, to work with a bereaved client. Bearing in mind that most people inevitably experience bereavement during their lives, that will probably be all of you. This book aims to help you feel prepared to confidently support a client regardless of whether they have experienced a bereavement in the past or more recently; whether they have been through the loss of someone who has led a good long life or have lost someone to a traumatic 'out-of-order' death.

Most of us, depending on our modality, had either little or no training in working with bereaved clients. With the odd exception, most courses don't seem to cover the important subject of grief on their curriculum. As a result, many practitioners feel out of their depth when confronted with a visibly grieving client. This grief may be hard to witness for an unprepared practitioner, who is more likely to feel uncomfortable if they don't have either personal or past clinical experience of their client's particular loss. This is especially true if that loss is, for example, of a child, a partner or anyone who died in tragic circumstances.

How you handle a grieving client is a responsibility that cannot – and should not – be taken lightly. There is so much that wellness practitioners can do to support their grieving clients effectively – if they are equipped to do so. If not, a client can be left feeling their loss has been dismissed, minimized or, in some cases, ignored as the practitioner moves to the next question on their list. This can potentially compound their pain, and they may feel reluctant to return for another session.

Supporting Your Grieving Client will cover the necessity of allowing your client to tell their story, if they need to, and to feel heard. Some practitioners feel bound by the structure of their consultation process, yet this may be the most helpful and healing form of 'treatment' at that particular moment. This book will explain how not all losses are the same and how grief can potentially affect the mind, body and spirit. It will also provide useful tools and resources you can utilize with your grieving client.

It's only in recent years that mental health issues have received the awareness and attention they deserve. I would like to see a similar improvement in awareness directed towards grief. Western society often shies away from the subject of death, and so it can feel stigmatized for those who are grieving. It may be that the Covid pandemic has started to change this to some extent. However, in view of both my experience and the experience of my grief coaching clients, it seems many people lack sensitivity towards, or understanding of, the complexity and far-reaching effects of a significant loss. The more grief-aware we can be, the more resilient grieving people can become. A grief-aware and compassionate practitioner has an opportunity to be at the forefront of this change.

The physical manifestations of grief are often overlooked by the conventional grief support on offer, and this is an area where you can really make a huge difference. Typically, some of your bereaved clients will visit their general practitioner (GP) for advice and may seek the support of a bereavement counsellor. It doesn't seem to be in the remit of most bereavement counsellors to discuss in any depth the physical symptoms, and GPs tend to just offer antidepressants or sleeping medication as their solution. Before my own experience, I had no idea that grief could be such a physical thing, so visceral. It can put tremendous strain on your body, and, as we will see, there is research to demonstrate how it can sometimes lead to very serious health issues, such as cancer and heart disease, if not addressed and supported. Your client could benefit from your knowledge and understanding of the physical aspects of grief, and this book aims to provide you with this so that you can confidently support them.

Supporting Your Grieving Client is intended for all professional wellness practitioners, including the following:

- acupuncturists
- Alexander technique practitioners
- aromatherapists
- Bowen therapists
- craniosacral therapists
- emotional freedom technique (EFT) practitioners
- healers
- herbalists
- homeopaths
- hypnotherapists
- massage therapists
- naturopaths
- neuro-linguistic programming (NLP) practitioners
- nutritional therapists
- reflexologists
- reiki practitioners
- shiatsu practitioners
- wellbeing and life coaches
- yoga therapists.

It is hoped that this book will be a useful addition to your bookshelf that you can refer to when you have a client who:

- has had a recent bereavement
- has lost a close family member, spouse or partner
- has experienced a traumatic loss – that is, a

sudden or 'out-of-order' death such as the loss of
a child, loss of a sibling, parent or partner who
is not elderly, loss of a grandchild
- has lost anyone to murder or suicide or has unexpectedly
  witnessed the dead body of someone known to them
- was separated and unable to say goodbye to their
  loved one – for example, during lockdown.

Practitioners of all types have an opportunity to make a significant difference to the healing journey of their grieving client. To do so, it will help not only to have a thorough understanding of the reality of grief but also to not be afraid to sit with your client's emotional pain, acknowledging that although your particular way of working may be well placed to support certain aspects of their healing, you cannot necessarily make it all better when it comes to grief. In some cases, the loss may be life-changing. Therefore, when you're supporting someone who is grieving, it's important to respect that you're not trying to get them 'back on track', as if their grief is just a temporary blip before they resume their old life; instead, your role is to support them as they navigate a new path. As Megan Devine says in her book *It's OK That You're Not OK: Meeting Grief and Loss in a Culture That Doesn't Understand*: 'Some things cannot be fixed. They can only be carried.'[1]

MY STORY

I began to practise as a CNHC- and BANT-registered nutritional therapist 15 years ago and then later as a wellbeing coach, too. The death of my son three years ago changed my life beyond measure, and once I eventually began working again after a year off, it changed the way I worked, too. I'm now a trauma-informed holistic grief coach, supporting clients in addressing all aspects of the grieving process

---

1   Devine, 2017, p.3

and how it can affect the body, as well as our emotional, mental and spiritual wellbeing. This addition to my practice came about because I couldn't find the grief support that I needed when first bereaved and knew others who didn't either. (I saw a bereavement counsellor, trauma therapist and several wellness practitioners.) Writing became my therapy, a way of processing what had happened to me. This eventually took the form of my book *Love Untethered: How to Live When Your Child Dies*.

My own profound loss revealed how little genuine compassion some of those working in mainstream medicine have towards the bereaved, but it also unfortunately highlighted for me how unenlightened some alternative health practitioners are when it comes to dealing with clients who are coping with grief. An example of this would be the practitioner I saw who compared the tragic, out-of-order death of my son with that of her cat and father, both of whom had led long lives, and told me dismissively that 'we've all lost children in past lives'. I saw another who was adamant she could relieve me of post-traumatic stress disorder (PTSD) using a little-known therapy, despite how, halfway through the (very expensive) package of sessions, I told her I wasn't feeling any discernible change whatsoever. They were well intentioned but misguided in their underestimation of the depth of my pain and trauma, and in their overconfidence that their particular skill set could help someone in such intense grief.

Unfortunately, during the writing of this book, I have experienced two further losses. First, my father passed away. This was a very different experience of grief for me when compared with the loss of my child. My dad was elderly, and his death was expected, and although I found it upsetting to witness some of the suffering that he experienced during the months leading up to his death, I took comfort from the fact that, unlike my son, he had lived a long life and that I had the opportunity to say goodbye. His death was not a shock but part of the natural order of life. It was therefore much easier to accept than the premature death of my child when every part of my being was irrevocably altered due to the sudden and brutal severing of this primal bond. The contrasting experiences of these two losses augmented my understanding of the undeniable diversity and complexity of grief.

A few days after my father's death, my husband tested positive for Covid, and, soon after, so did I, which meant I was unable to go to my father's funeral. Far worse was to come. Shockingly, just three weeks after the death of my father, I lost my husband, too. Once again, my life was thrown into complete turmoil by another traumatic loss, triggering the PTSD I experienced after my son's death. I was unable to visit my husband until he was dying because I was ill myself, and because no visitors were permitted to the Covid ward anyway. This added to my anguish, as it undoubtedly would have done for many of the bereaved who lost a loved one during the pandemic. However, I was allowed to be with him (in full PPE) as he died. This was an utterly harrowing experience, but it was also a privilege to be with him as he crossed over to be reunited with our son.

Both the fallout caused by losing someone during the pandemic and the effect that profound grief potentially has on increasing inflammation and suppressing immunity will be covered later in the book. My husband had no underlying health conditions, was not overweight, had a healthy diet and lifestyle, took supplements, etc. He was, however, a bereaved father...

As you will now understand, my own experience of loss and trauma has informed how I work with my clients, and, through this book, I aim to share my knowledge, which has evolved from both personal and professional experience. By doing so, I hope to help other practitioners, like you, to become more grief-aware and better informed, and to not over-promise, due to an underestimation of the life-shattering effect of some bereavements. These clients need to be handled with care and sensitivity, but if you are able to make an appreciable difference to their healing, then they can be very rewarding to work with. So thank you for picking up this book and being a practitioner who is willing to develop their understanding of this important issue.

CHAPTER 1

Types of Grief

This chapter will address the different types of grief and the fact that not all grief is exactly the same. Every relationship is unique, so inevitably every experience of grief is also going to be unique. One person who has lost their mother is not going to feel exactly the same as their friend who also lost their mother. It will depend on their relationship with them (whether predominantly positive or negative) as well as their individual level of resilience. It can also depend on how their loved one died and whether it was peaceful or involved a great deal of suffering, whether it was expected or unexpected. Whether it was a long life or a life cut short will also affect the grief. Tolerance to emotional pain can vary enormously in a griever. A highly sensitive person may cope less well with a loss than someone with a more robust nature.

Grief can be brutal. It can be enormously complex, and its path and reach of pain can be surprising and unpredictable, so it's best to never make assumptions about how it might feel for your client. Grief expert David Kessler[1] says the worst loss is your loss, and this is, of course, inevitably true. Because every relationship we have in life is different, and therefore each loss is experienced differently, some people will undoubtedly cope better than others. It's important, then, for us as practitioners not to make assumptions or compare

---

1   Kessler, 2019

our client's grief with our own experience of loss. We also need to be mindful of bringing any personal views on death, or what we believe happens after death, into play – at least until we have learned more about our client's beliefs on the subject. Something else to bear in mind is that bereaved people report feeling judged if they are perceived to be coping well, yet also if they don't appear to be 'getting over' their loss. It's important therefore to accept someone where they are and however they may feel.

Comparing grief is a contentious topic but it's likely that you may find a vast difference in the intensity of grief, and its physical and emotional ramifications, between someone who has lost an elderly relative and someone who has lost a child, for example. My observation (as well as my own personal experience) has been that the grief for someone who has had an acceptable lifespan has a natural progression where the sadness of the loss usually lessens over time. By contrast, losing someone who has died at a young age, or tragically in any way, will invariably need a greater level of support, and working with them is inevitably challenging because the loss is so life-changing. In the words of Joseph P. Kennedy: 'When the young bury the old, time heals the pain and sorrow. But when the process is reversed, the sorrow remains forever.'[2] These grievers are never going to 'get over' their loss. However, helping these clients find measurable ways to support themselves through the worst of all losses and ease some of their suffering can be especially rewarding.

These are the types of grief you could see in your clinic.

NORMAL GRIEF

You could argue about what's 'normal', but, in the context of grief, it's probably along the lines of (1) a reaction to a loss that doesn't throw someone completely off balance; (2) sorrow that gradually diminishes over time; and (3) the ability to engage in normal daily

---

2   Renehan, 2002, Chapter 28

activities again relatively quickly. In other words, although sad, the loss wasn't traumatic or dramatically life-changing. Normal grief is more likely to occur if the person who died had a normal lifespan and the death was expected, or if the relationship was not that close.

ANTICIPATORY GRIEF

This may happen when someone watches their loved one die over a period of time, whether that happens to be weeks or months. The griever understands that the person is going to die and begins to grieve before the person has actually passed away. Aside from watching someone die from a long-term physical illness, such as cancer, anticipatory grief can also be experienced when there is mental illness or dementia, or in any case when someone doesn't have the mental capacity or awareness that they used to have. It is painful to witness personality changes as these usually result in changes of interaction and a hard-to-witness disintegration of how the relationship once was. There may be grief at the powerlessness of not being able to change things, not being able to make things better for the loved one, and an inability to help them get back to who they once were.

If you see someone who is facing anticipatory grief for whatever reason, then the ongoing stress they experience in this situation can very much be supported and eased by alternative and complementary therapies. They may be on 'high alert' as they wait for the dreaded phone call from the hospital, and this can take its toll, affecting sleep and eating and just generally raising levels of anxiety as they wait for their loved one to die. Anticipatory grief can offer a certain amount of preparation for what's to come and gives the opportunity to leave nothing unsaid, which can, in some cases, mean less chance of the grief becoming 'complicated' later on. It may still, however, be a very difficult experience.

DELAYED GRIEF

This can occur if the bereaved person becomes preoccupied with something other than actually living with the stark reality of their loss. This can include a fight for justice if, for example, the person who died was killed in a hit-and-run accident. The bereaved person may distract themselves from feeling the full extent of the pain while focusing on something else, even if that something else is related to the person who has died.

Waiting for an inquest may also delay grief. Some may find they put their grief on hold until they have got through this additional ordeal. This can be a tortuous time as inquests happen when circumstances are unexplained and the death is unexpected. Depending where you live, the wait for an inquest can be months, or even years sometimes, and waiting to be informed of the date only adds to the excruciating anxiety.

The distraction of having to sort through practical matters for someone who left their affairs in disarray can also delay grief. If the bereaved person can't find a will or get into the phone or access the email of the person who has died, or they don't know who they banked with or what utility or car insurance companies they used, for example, it can get very stressful and overwhelming. They may find they have no space yet – or indeed time or energy – to really feel the actual pain of loss.

Another example of delayed grief would be a mother who loses her husband and has to maintain a level of normalcy and practicality for the sake of their children. Although this can help to pace out the loss to some extent, it can be an enormous strain to constantly pretend – and feel totally exhausting to keep this up. The grief may be delayed for quite some time, often until the children are older and more self-sufficient. A parent's instinct is usually to put their children first, regardless of what they themselves are coping with.

And sometimes the force of someone's grief is just too much to bear, so it is delayed until a later date when their brain deems it 'safe' to process. This can sometimes take years, and another loss or traumatic incident may serve as a trigger.

COMPLICATED GRIEF

This tends to be long-term and will frequently be seen with an out-of-order death when someone has died before their time, and/or suddenly and unexpectedly, and/or through suicide or murder. It is also quite likely to happen when there have been multiple losses, especially if these have occurred in a relatively short time frame. There may well be trauma and possibly a diagnosis of PTSD associated with complicated grief. Emotional and physical symptoms may be seen to be debilitating and long-lasting, impairing the ability to function normally, whether socially, at work or with simple everyday tasks. You may observe depression and anxiety if you see a client with complicated grief, as well as suicidal ideation. You may need to refer on or work in conjunction alongside an experienced grief practitioner.

TRAUMATIC GRIEF

Day-to-day functioning can be disrupted as a person struggles to cope with the enormous shock of losing someone who died suddenly, violently, with a great deal of suffering or at a young age. Bereaved parents invariably experience traumatic grief and again, this is often accompanied by a diagnosis of PTSD. There are crossovers with complicated grief and the terms are sometimes used interchangeably.

CUMULATIVE GRIEF

This can happen when a subsequent loss (or losses) occurs during the time that someone is still in the midst of grieving the first. This can lead to a system overload and a feeling of being totally engulfed by seemingly intolerable grief. Sometimes it's too much, and any additional losses cannot be fully processed so they get put on hold, become merged or are simply never fully experienced. The effect of cumulative grief due to multiple losses can also result in excessive fear and anxiety around losing more loved ones – this will no longer seem beyond the realm of possibility when you've lost more than one person.

Using my own experience to illustrate, when my father died, I was not only still grieving my son, but I was also ill with Covid, unable to go to my father's funeral, and my husband was in hospital. I imagined I would come back to 'processing' what his loss meant to me, although I knew, in contrast with my son's loss, it was unlikely to stop me from functioning. However, when my husband died, the impact and devastation of this loss superseded the loss of my father (but not that of my child), and I was unable to grieve my dad any further. However, I was still left with two very major losses to deal with. This situation can lead to grief feeling confused – who is this pain of loss for? If the losses are from the same family, as in my case of a son and a husband, perhaps that feeling is inevitable. Feelings can at times seem to merge together in a big pool of grief, and at other times they feel more distinct.

Although my losses were close in terms of time frame, and two of them were traumatic, it may seem that I'm an extreme example – and I am. However, it's quite likely that you will come across clients who have had multiple losses in a more extended time frame but who are definitely still experiencing a form of cumulative grief. An example, perhaps more typical than my own story, is a client I had who had lost her father to cancer when she was 16, a close friend in a car crash at 22 and, during the time I was working with her, a miscarriage at 17 weeks when she was 31. The miscarriage very much triggered the pain of the previous losses, which had not been fully processed at the time they happened.

CHRONIC GRIEF

It might be easy to assume chronic grief sounds unhealthy, but if someone has experienced a life-shattering loss (or more than one), their grief is inevitably going to be long-term and its intensity on-going. Many people who have experienced a profound loss (or losses) eventually accept that their grief will be forever, as they move from acute grief to chronic grief. It's still possible, however, to live a life with some purpose and meaning alongside long-term and ongoing chronic grief. This is far from ideal, obviously, and very sad, but it's important to understand that this may be the best it will get for some people. It's crucial not to tell them: 'It will get better.' You don't know that. That's not to say that it *won't* get better, but those experiencing this type of grief frequently feel others don't fully grasp the magnitude of what's happened to them or how insurmountable their situation feels. This comment might confirm that view.

In this type of grief, the pain of loss can actually feel worse in some ways as time goes on. The assumption is that all grief will gradually improve, especially after the first year. This is far from true in certain cases. There is no time frame for grief and, although every person is different, in the case of a profound loss, the second and third years, and even beyond, are often reported to be worse that the first, usually because the shock of what's happened gradually wears off and the raw pain underneath is revealed. If several losses are endured, then the period of intense grief is potentially extended even further. It's very important to understand that some grief can last a lifetime.

PROLONGED GRIEF

The difference between chronic grief, complicated grief and prolonged grief looks, on the face of it, to be splitting hairs. However, 'prolonged grief' is recognized as a distinct psychiatric disorder according to the updated 2022 version of the *Diagnostic and Statistical Manual of Mental Disorders* (DSM-5).[3] Prolonged grief disorder is classed as intense grief that lasts beyond a year. This is controversial to say the least, and respected grief experts such as Megan Devine and David Kessler recognize that grief is highly individual, has no time limit and is not a 'disorder' but a natural response to having loved someone deeply. I don't know of a single bereaved parent whose grief

---

3   APA, 2022

isn't still very intense after just a year! Yet prolonged grief disorder is now considered to be a mental illness. Although it's argued that a diagnosis could offer some sort of acknowledgement and validation to the griever, it is basically labelling grief felt beyond a designated time period as a mental disorder, and there are concerns that this will inevitably be deemed to automatically necessitate medication. Many feel strongly that grief shouldn't be categorized in this way, that it creates a stigma and sets us back in our understanding of what is, in some cases, the long-term impact of death. Some losses will naturally be felt powerfully for much longer than the 'allowed' 12 months, and Megan Devine, among others, says that pathologizing grief in this way can be damaging, contributing to a feeling of shame for grieving the 'wrong way' and for too long.

(I should add that the *Diagnostic and Statistical Manual of Mental Disorders* (DSM-5) is an American publication, so its main impact will be in the US, where clinicians use the DSM-5 to diagnose mental disorders. Clinicians in the UK predominantly use the ICD-10 system to diagnose mental disorders, while the DSM classification system is mostly used for research purposes. However, as is often the case, what happens in the US influences opinion and protocols worldwide.)

DISENFRANCHISED GRIEF

Disenfranchised grief – also known as hidden grief – can be experienced when grief goes unsupported and unacknowledged, and feels invalidated in some way. This may be because it is considered by others as somehow unworthy, not valid, not significant, or is associated with a stigma. Disenfranchised grief can sometimes be seen in cases where the relationship was LGBTQ+ (if family or friends don't accept the sexuality of the person who died, same-sex partners can feel excluded from the grieving process); with an ex-partner or spouse; with the death of an estranged family member; a step-parent or step- or half-sibling; when partners weren't married; or when someone has had an affair with the person who has died. Disenfranchised grief can also be experienced with miscarriage, which is often shockingly unsupported, and in cases of abortion, too. It can be felt whenever there may be any kind of social stigma, such as death from addiction, overdose or suicide. Bereaved people experience significantly less support or sympathy when a death is associated with mental illness, addiction or an overdose in comparison to those whose loved one died because of a physical illness, such as cancer. When society fails to acknowledge these types of losses, it makes it challenging for the bereaved person to express their grief, potentially silencing and shaming them.

COLLECTIVE GRIEF

This is grief experienced by a society or community as the result of something like a natural disaster, terrorist attack or death of a public figure. One unique issue with collective grief is that the families who have lost someone to this type of event can feel that their individual loss is overshadowed by being one of several (or many) losses, as well as by people's outpouring of collective grief towards someone they didn't actually know, which may spark feelings of anger in the bereaved family or friends.

Many people find themselves taken by surprise at their depth of emotion for a public figure that they have never actually met. The death of Princess Diana is a good example of this and, more recently, the Queen. In contrast to the outpouring of emotion expressed for the tragic death of Princess Diana, those who queued for many hours to see the Queen's coffin were generally observed to be doing so to show their respect and gratitude for her life of service.

Collective grief can facilitate a positive connection with others through the ritual of public mourning. It is often granted more free-dom of expression than private grief and some may feel more able to grieve openly and without judgement. (By contrast, this is not always everyone's experience of sharing their personal grief.) Everyone is reminded of their own experiences of loss and, in some cases, this can prove cathartic. However, for many recently bereaved, or with experience of profound grief, the extensive and inescapable media coverage of national mourning for the Queen felt overwhelmingly relentless. For some coping with a tragic loss, there was a feeling of resentment towards the considerable attention devoted to a woman who was fortunate to have lived a full and very long life, not to mention a privileged one. Overall, our experience of collective grief will undoubtedly be shaped by our personal circumstances.

ABSENT GRIEF

Sometimes people might not seem to be grieving at all, or at least not as much as society deems that they 'should'. It's easy to assume they're in denial or that their grief will hit them later on, but some bereaved people may just feel underwhelmed after a loss, with anticipated emotions being far less than they had imagined. This is not always recognized, or indeed considered acceptable, so there may be guilt or even shame around not feeling enough. It's obviously important not to judge someone who doesn't appear to be experiencing grief for their loss. Everyone grieves differently, and there may be many different reasons why absent grief occurs. It may be due to numbness or dissociation, in which case the grief will probably resurface at a later date, but it could also be due to a lack of closeness to the person who died (even if they were a close family member), not seeing them for a long time, already having experienced anticipatory grief, or simply because the bereaved person is innately resilient by nature.

LOCKDOWN GRIEF

This is obviously a new type of grief. The Covid lockdowns have meant that there have been many cases of people being physically unable to be with their dying loved ones when they might ordinarily have had the opportunity to do so. This inevitably can lead to complicated feelings. There may be anger, helplessness or guilt at not being allowed to visit during the illness or to be there at someone's final moments in life. In addition, and compounding these feelings, many were unable to hold proper funerals and gather friends and family together to formally say goodbye in this traditional rite of passage. Grief is an isolating experience at the best of times, but this became magnified at the height of the pandemic – not only because friends and family could not physically be there to comfort the bereaved, but because it was a time when everyone was preoccupied with fears about their own mortality. In addition, those bereaved by non-Covid losses during this time may have felt their grief was overshadowed by those who have lost someone to Covid.

All of the above could lead to complicated loss. In the study 'Loss and grief amidst COVID-19: A path to adaption and resilience', the researchers concluded:

> Loss, as a more encompassing theme, interweaves many aspects of people's life in this challenging time. Failure to address the pressing needs of those experiencing loss and grief may result in poor mental and physical health. Recognizing the uniqueness of each individual and their loss and grief will provide opportunities to develop tailored strategies that facilitate functional adaptation to loss and promote mental health and wellbeing in this crisis.[4]

SECONDARY LOSSES

It's really crucial to be mindful that your client may encounter a number of secondary losses that could seriously impact their life further. Secondary losses are often overlooked, but your client could be experiencing any of the following, depending on the type of loss.

---

4   Zhai and Du, 2020, p.80

Loss of a future

If they've lost a child or a partner, a bereaved person can feel they don't have a future to look forward to any more. They grieve what could have been and for all the hopes and plans they had. If a child has died, the parents have to witness their child's friends reaching milestones their child won't, such as significant birthdays, graduation, getting married, having children, etc. When a partner has died, there is a loss of companionship. Not having someone to share everyday life with, or holidays or significant dates, will inevitably feel very sad, not to mention lonely. Younger bereaved partners may meet someone else in time, but many in their middle years or older may face the prospect of countless years alone, and that could feel daunting for them.

Loss of their past

This happens when someone loses a parent, sibling or childhood friend – someone who has, up until now, always been part of their lives. They shared their entire past with that person. Young adults, in particular, can find this difficult to cope with. For children of all ages, their world can now feel unsafe, and they wonder who they might lose next. Older children who have lost siblings may decide they don't want to have children of their own for fear of going through what they've witnessed their parents going through.

Loss of identity

Who are they if they're no longer a mother or wife, for example? Our perception of who we are is integral to our sense of wellbeing. Coaches can help here, perhaps (when the time is right) encouraging a grieving client to explore other aspects of themselves.

Loss of financial security

If someone loses a partner whose income was essential, this can put grief on hold while practicalities are addressed and can add to anxiety and a lack of feeling safe. This can precipitate anger at their loved one for leaving them to deal with this additional worry. A reduced household income may necessitate a return to work before the griever feels ready and may also precipitate a change in lifestyle (in spending habits generally, including the food they buy, holidays, treats, subscriptions, repairs or replacements of household items, heating the home, etc.) in order to accommodate their new financial circumstances. In some cases, it can even mean selling their home. To experience these unwanted changes in addition to the loss itself feels grossly unfair and can greatly exacerbate their stress, impacting their grief further.

Loss of friendships

Lack of support from friends is a very common experience in cases of child or partner loss and comes as a surprise to many. These particular losses are most people's worst nightmare and so they may avoid the bereaved due to their own fear of death and loss. Loss of friendships is also common in young people whose peers may not have the life experience or maturity to support their friend who has perhaps lost a parent or sibling and understand their ensuing difficult emotions. Often people just don't know what to say; instead, they make the choice to avoid someone who is grieving so they don't have to feel uncomfortable. From the point of view of the griever, this is very hurtful, exacerbating their pain and sense of isolation.

Loss of career

This may happen if someone's grief, shock, PTSD or depression leaves them unable to work or they lose their job because they need to take time off. As a result, they may experience loss of income and loss of identity, too. This can feel very demoralizing and potentially precipitate further spiralling. After a profound loss, it's sometimes a case of not being able to go back to their 'before' life when their person was still alive. It can feel as though it's somehow wrong to go back to what you once did when you now inhabit such a different world. I lost all my clients when I was incapable of working after my son's death, and I didn't work for nearly a year. In the latter part of that time, I decided I would find another way of working that could incorporate my new world, and so I made the decision to start practising as a holistic grief coach, assimilating both my 'before' and 'after' skills, with my extended reading and study on the subject of grief and trauma. Taking time out, restructuring or changing a career in order to go forward differently into their post-loss world might not be possible for everyone. In fact, this wasn't the case for me either after my husband died as, without his income, I had to go back to work much sooner than I would have liked. However, it might be worth exploring any new ways your client could move forward with their work life in order to reflect their changed circumstances, as this could potentially inspire a glimmer of hope for their future.

Loss of family structure

The death of a family member can have a devastating effect upon the family dynamic. It impacts family occasions such as birthdays, weddings, celebrations, family holidays, etc. The death of a parent within a family structure means the remaining parent has to take on extra responsibilities, as well as dealing with their own grief. The death of a child means that the remaining sibling(s) will change position within the family, now becoming, for instance, the only child, the eldest or the youngest. The loss of the original family structure and dynamic is very destabilizing for all concerned, and its momentous impact as a secondary loss should not be underestimated. In addition, after the initial shock waves have dissipated, the family may not necessarily grieve together as a unit. In many cases, because each member of a family will grieve in disparate ways, it can feel as if relationships are fractured and everyone is on a different page.

Loss of a marriage or partnership

Marriages and partnerships can certainly be adversely affected by grief, too. When one partner is grieving and the other isn't, it can impact the relationship. The non-grieving partner may become impatient, wondering why their partner is grieving beyond the time frame that they feel is appropriate for the loss of a parent, sibling or friend. This can lead to the grieving partner feeling let down or abandoned. The relationship between bereaved parents can also be affected despite their shared loss, and there are some statistics floating around which suggest divorce rates among bereaved parents are up to 80 per cent. However, in a 2006 study commissioned by The Compassionate Friends, parental divorce following the death of a child was found to be significantly less than that, at around 16 per cent.[5]

Loss of stability

This can affect many types of grievers but may be felt particularly with young people who experience the loss of a parent or sibling. Not only do they have their own grief to cope with but they also have to witness the pain of their parents' grief, too. This can be very frightening. Their life has already changed beyond recognition, and in addition they have their stability further shattered by seeing the parent(s) they depend on for a sense of security appearing very vulnerable and seemingly no longer able to provide a sense of stability. Widows (and no doubt widowers too) also report feeling a loss of stability – their partner may have provided a feeling of safety and security that they took for granted when they were still alive.

---

5   Frogge, 2015

Feeling safe, stable and secure are seen as essential components for good mental health.

Loss of confidence

Grief, especially if the loss was unexpected, can make your client feel very vulnerable and shake their self-esteem. They can suddenly feel very unsafe in a world where they now know from experience anything can happen. Everything they thought to be true is thrown into question. Building back self-esteem is another good area for coaches to work in and make a difference.

As you can see, grief is varied and complex and highly individual, dependent on a vast array of factors. The more you are aware of this, the more you can demonstrate an understanding of your client, share any of the information found here that might help them to process their current situation, and tailor your therapy/treatment sessions accordingly.

(Although experiencing the death of a parent as a child is a loss you may certainly come across, the trauma of which may still be having an impact, it is assumed here that your clients are adults, rather than children under the age of 18. In addition, you will no doubt see clients going through other sorts of grief, such as loss of a pet, divorce or loss of a job, to name a few. These can all be challenging and affect us in a myriad of ways, but for the purposes of this book, we are looking at the effect that losing another human being has upon someone's emotional, physical and spiritual wellbeing.)

CHAPTER 2

The Skills Most Needed

The most important qualities you need for a grieving client are compassion and being a good listener, without feeling the need to give your opinion on their experience of grief. Aim to be of service in this way and, although there's a place for both compassion *and* strategy, let go of jumping straight in with what you think will help, certainly initially. Tools that you use with non-grieving clients may not work with grieving ones. It may be judicious when sitting in the presence of someone's raw grief to abandon your questionnaire or usual treatment temporarily, in order to prioritize allowing a client to feel properly heard. (Grievers frequently report that they don't feel that they are.) This can sometimes provide more effective 'pain relief' than any of the other tools you may have in the toolkit. As David Kessler has said: 'Loss can be more meaningful – and more bearable – when reflected, and reflected accurately, in another's eyes.'[1]

If you haven't been in practice long, not following, to the letter, the way you have been taught to do things can feel a little scary. However, being adaptable and using your intuition as you navigate a session is pretty much up there with good listening skills and compassion if you really want to help someone who is grieving. Even though a client might have come to you for a physical symptom, if they start to open up or get emotional about their grief, please allow

---

1   Kessler, 2019, p.33

them the space to do so. It really will potentially be as beneficial as anything else you can do for them.

If you already know they have experienced a bereavement that is either significant and/or recent, you could perhaps send out any questionnaire in advance (if you don't already do this). That way, you could free up some of the consultation time. If that's not an option or you don't know in advance about their loss, and the usual course of your session doesn't get to what you might normally cover, you can always explain at the end that you thought it more important to give them the space to talk about their loss. Then perhaps send some questions you didn't get to ask and/or some simple well-considered advice in an email afterwards, and explain how in their next session you will get going on your usual treatment or therapy, tailored to their current situation.

It is an important part of the healing process for grief to be witnessed and validated. If they trust you enough to open up about their emotional pain, then you are most likely successfully building a rapport with them. Your treatment/protocol will also now be better informed by hearing about their experience of loss and how it's affecting them. You may also be able to join some dots that they haven't, such as how a flare-up of irritable bowel syndrome (IBS) could be related to their grief. It's also good to remember that any information you go on to give them will be assimilated more effectively when your client feels safe, so building trust and rapport is key for compliance.

It may be that a client comes to you with grief as their main issue, or it may that they will come for something else and that you will then see that their grief is an 'underlying cause'. In some cases, if it's a profound and/or recent loss, this will be front and centre of how you go on to support them. However, it may be that grief isn't part of the reason they've come to see you, but enquiry into their family history inadvertently prompts floods of tears as they tell you about their father's recent death or how their little brother died of cancer aged 12.

Often with women, it's when you're asking about children and pregnancies that it comes to light that they have had miscarriages, an abortion or a stillborn baby. This obviously needs to be handled with great sensitivity as very often, after a relatively short period of time, these particular losses are barely referred to again by those around them, especially if the woman then goes on to have other children. You may find that giving them the opportunity to talk about what happened proves cathartic and that they may leave the session feeling lighter as a result of you giving them the space to share their loss with you.

As a nutritional therapist, before my own bereavements (i.e. before I knew better), I would generally offer a few sympathetic words when someone got a bit tearful as I asked about their family history, but I was usually quite keen to move on to my next question, mindful of all I wanted to get through during the consultation. If your client seems okay to move on, then, by all means, do so, but if this has in any way 'unlocked' something in them, it really is better to allow them to express whatever your question has prompted. Ultimately, we want to support our clients in their healing in whatever way possible, so if this is coming unexpectedly from left field, just go with it. Even if you're not a conventional therapist or counsellor you can still, within your remit, offer very valuable emotional as well as physical support which many will appreciate. Approaching grief from our holistic perspective, and especially where there is trauma, has so much to offer.

The above examples centre around grief presenting as possibly 'incidental' to the reason someone has come to see you. However, it's likely that, sooner or later, you will see someone in the midst of early grief – classed, incidentally, by David Kessler[2] as the first two years and by The Compassionate Friends, the charity for bereaved parents,[3] as five years in cases of child loss. This might be a much longer time

---

2   Kessler, n.d.
3   https://www.compassionatefriends.org

frame than you may have assumed. Surviving early grief and just getting through the day can take supreme effort if the loss is being felt very keenly. There is simply no time limit on grief; everyone is very different, and, for some, grief is lifelong. As Joanne Cacciatore (author of *Bearing the Unbearable*) is quoted as saying, if you can't understand why someone is grieving so much, and for so long, then consider yourself fortunate that you don't understand.

Clients in the early stages may have come specifically to see you about a matter directly related to their grief. These symptoms could typically include insomnia, anxiety, depression, brain fog, fatigue, digestive issues, headaches, hormonal issues. These are all issues you probably see every day (depending on any specialism you might have), but now you may possibly have a specific underlying cause, and that is the emotional impact of grief.

Although you may feel more comfortable focusing mainly on the symptoms, rather than the root cause of them, it's quite possible that during the course of a consultation you will come face to face with your client's raw grief, especially if they're quite early on in the grieving process – and that may feel daunting if you don't have much personal or clinical experience of this. Do your very best to let go of your own discomfort or any need to 'make it better'. Don't be afraid of just allowing them to be sad. Let them tell their story if that's what would benefit them most – that's all you have to do for now. Again, the importance of enabling your client to feel heard cannot be over-emphasized. It's surprising how many bereaved people are made to feel their emotions around grief are inconvenient in some way. They'll be so pleased if you don't make them feel like this.

A little about what your grieving client may be experiencing from other people's reaction to their grief and why, consequently, they may be watchful of how you respond. There is sadly often an implication that someone who is grieving has a responsibility to hide their pain in case it upsets others and makes them feel uncomfortable. The bereaved frequently feel pressurized into making their grief in some way more palatable for others.

Being in the presence of someone who has experienced a profound loss seems sometimes to manifest in others as either patronizing pity (usually with a half-smile and a head tilt) or else a fear response. I have lost count of the bereaved mothers I've spoken to who relate stories of people they know pretending not to have seen them or literally crossing the road to avoid them. As Megan Devine comments in her book *It's OK That You're Not OK*,[4] we are the stuff of other people's nightmares. Our culture generally does not handle grief well, especially when it's confronted with most people's idea of the worst thing that can happen in life, such as losing a child or spouse or having a family member who was murdered or took their own life. As if what they're going through isn't bad enough, these bereaved people can end up feeling very stigmatized and isolated as a result of other people's inability to deal with their fears around death and their own mortality.

Even if you don't come across these more extreme losses, bear in mind that your grieving client may well have not always encountered an understanding or compassionate response, whatever the type of loss may be. They will almost certainly have encountered the expectation that they should be 'over it' within a certain time frame – and they really may not be. Society will often ignore, minimize, invalidate or dismiss the feelings of those who have experienced a loss. Unfortunately, grief is not a choice, it's not optional, yet there often appears to be an implication that grief should be hidden, especially after the first few weeks, because it's simply unpalatable for others to witness. If you are aware of all of the above, and how your client may have been made to feel, you'll be in a better place to hold space for them, making clear that whatever they feel is okay. This not only demonstrates kindness and compassion; it helps to build their trust and confidence in your ability to help them.

If you feel there's a need to ask a question at this stage, please never let it be 'How did they die?' This is so intrusive. They may well

---

4   Devine, 2017

tell you and that's fine, but once you've found out who it is they've lost, your best first question is 'What were they like?' I can't emphasize enough how everyone is likely to really appreciate this question, and it gives you a chance to humanize their loss. You may be keen to know if there's a family history of cancer or heart disease, in case this provides you with useful information on how to treat them, but you can find this out later. Where there is trauma around the circumstances of a death, it's essential not to go there until the client is ready and you have established a relationship and built up trust and a feeling of safely for them. To disregard this and to dive in with such an insensitive question would be highly irresponsible.

It's always best not to give your opinion on what they tell you about the person who died, their death or how your client might be feeling now or in the future. You may consider their loved one to be at peace now after fighting a lengthy cancer 'battle', but maybe your grieving client doesn't see it that way. If someone caused your client huge long-term stress due to mental health issues and made suicide attempts before actually ending their life, your client still might not have been prepared for this shock and most likely may not feel relieved not to have to worry about that person any more. Please remember that time does not heal *all* wounds. In Chapter 7, we will go into more detail about what to say and what not to say. It can feel like a bit of a minefield, but you will eventually feel confident that what you say will help and not hinder.

A note for coaches and NLP practitioners: we're often on the lookout for limiting beliefs being expressed by our clients and how these may be holding them back. You may hear a lot of what you perceive to be limiting beliefs in your grieving client, such as 'I will never get over this', 'Why did this happen to me?', 'I should have been a better daughter/mother/friend/husband', 'If only I had...', 'I'm not sure I can go on without her'. If they have lost a very significant person, allow them to feel all of this. They're experiencing a normal response to loss, and, in fact, the best thing you can do is reassure them of this. Do not help them to reframe their belief, however negative it may sound to you. Coaching a grieving client is very different from coaching our other clients. In some cases, the grieving client will gradually work through these beliefs for themselves, as they begin to accommodate their loss into their life and feel more hopeful, and they may even use your sessions to do so. In others, though, these beliefs may remain pretty much in place. It is never our place to judge that someone who has had a life-altering loss is somehow 'stuck' in their grief and to view this as negative and in need of changing. Unless you have walked in their shoes – and even if you have – respect their feelings and don't try to fix their thinking.

As coaches, we are also inherently goal-focused, and again this is not very appropriate during grief, especially in the early stages when survival isn't about achievement, looking towards the future, trying to find something that will inspire or light you up or give you a reason for living. For some, it may literally be about getting through the day, hour by hour, minute by minute. In normal coaching circumstances, there is value in cheerleading a client, but you simply can't cheerlead anyone out of deep grief. Someone who has experienced a traumatic loss is highly unlikely to resonate with the pursuit of happiness or success – this may now feel completely alien to them, and they are more likely to just want to find a little peace.

Most people who are drawn to helping others are empathic and compassionate, so you are likely to have these much-needed qualities naturally when it comes to working with someone who is grieving. Compassion, good listening skills, following your intuition and remaining adaptable during your consultations are the skills you can hone to successfully support your grieving client. Then all you need to do is develop your awareness of how grief actually feels for them, without making any assumptions, and how it may be manifesting in the mind, body and spirit.

CHAPTER 3

Physical Manifestations of Grief

As Irish writer and scholar C.S. Lewis said:

> No one ever told me that grief felt so like fear. I am not afraid, but the sensation is like being afraid. The same fluttering in the stomach, the same restlessness, the yawning. I keep on swallowing. At other times it feels like being mildly drunk, or concussed. There is a sort of invisible blanket between the world and me. I find it hard to take in what anyone says.[1]

Addressing the physical manifestations of grief is where many of you will be able to make a measurable difference to the healing of your grieving client. Most of us look at our clients from a holistic viewpoint, making connections between how their emotions might be getting expressed through their bodies. Nowhere can this be seen more clearly than in grief and trauma. Grief and trauma can potentially wreak untold havoc on the physical health of our grieving clients.

---

1   Lewis, 2013, p.3

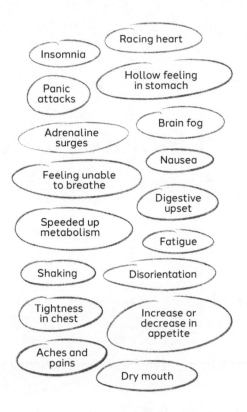

PHYSICAL MANIFESTATIONS OF GRIEF

Depending on the intensity of the grief, and the degree of trauma involved, your client may experience some or all of the above. Yet many of these bereaved clients could be surprised by this, because it's common to think of grief as causing predominantly emotional discomfort rather than physical discomfort in addition. One grief coaching client I worked with described the physicality of her grief as akin to being run over by a double-decker bus; another told me her brain felt as though it was swollen and stuffed with cotton wool. I was certainly very naïve about how grief might feel physically. It had never crossed my mind that there could be such powerful and extensive physical symptoms of grief, despite prior understanding of the link between mind, body and spirit. Here's how I described my own physical response to grief in my book *Love Untethered*:

I was amazed at the very extreme response my body had to the trauma of my son's sudden death. It reacted with violent shaking, a racing heart, a speeded-up metabolism, nausea, insomnia, a gnawing in the stomach and constantly catching my breath. All these symptoms were felt with great intensity and were ongoing for quite some time, which was both startling and overwhelming. This is shock. The nervous system goes into overdrive and the stress hormones, adrenaline and cortisol, are released as part of the fight or flight response because the body thinks it's in danger. Shock is fundamentally a protective mechanism and it stops you from having to deal with the full impact of the emotional trauma you're experiencing. The physical symptoms can temporarily distract from this, at least some of the time.[2]

Of course, not everyone experiences this level of physical reaction, but if there is shock involved, then it's quite possible some of these symptoms will occur and so it may therefore be well worth enquiring about whether they are, or have been, present. The more information you can gather about this, the more you can help your client. If someone is still experiencing these symptoms to the full, then it's quite possible they may feel they simply can't survive them. They will, but there may be a cost. During the first few months of grief, I didn't think I could possibly live another day without sleep, without being able to eat, with legs that seemed unable to hold me up, with my heart continually thumping out of my chest and literally hurting. Later on, there can be panic attacks, crippling fatigue, breathlessness, brain fog, not to mention endless, exhausting bouts of crying. Grief can be hugely debilitating. As I will outline in this chapter, based on research undertaken in this area, it is also capable of causing some serious longer-term damage to the body.

Like other major stressors, grief has the ability to affect the endocrine, immune, nervous, digestive and cardiovascular systems. It can

---

2   May, 2022, p.127

increase inflammation in the body quite dramatically, as we will see. An article in *Psychosomatic Medicine* reviewed the research undertaken since 1977 on the immune system's role in bereavement and concluded that 'a handful of recent good-quality studies show bereaved people demonstrate higher levels of systemic inflammation [and] maladaptive immune cell gene expression...compared with nonbereaved controls'.[3]

According to Psych Central, if someone had a physical illness before their loved one died, grief can exacerbate the existing illness. In addition, it can also open the way for a new physical illness, despite the fact that they may have been healthy prior to the loss. The bereaved can become more susceptible to minor illnesses such as sore throats and colds, as well more serious issues such as ulcerative colitis, rheumatoid arthritis, asthma, heart disease and cancer, which have all been shown to be connected to the stress of grief:

> The connection between the mind and body is not always recognized, but there is real scientific evidence that what we think and feel has a direct effect on our biological systems. This is an especially important issue for bereaved parents because the loss of a child is the ultimate in stress and a stress that lasts so very long.[4]

The physical expressions of grief that you might observe in your client give you an opportunity to do some really important damage limitation, and your grieving client will therefore be fortunate to have you to work with. Before I come on to some interesting scientific studies, I wanted to share with you an anecdotal one – these, as we know, can also be of value. In my bereaved parents' group of around 15 people, four of us have had cancer after the death of our child, one has developed Parkinson's disease, one had a heart attack and sadly two have died from Covid. When I heard the news that one of the bereaved mothers had died from Covid, I remember speculating that she probably died, at least in part, from a broken

---

3   Knowles, Ruiz and O'Connor, 2019, p.415
4   Pedersen, 2022

heart. Little did I know then that a year later my husband would also die this same way...

One of the more prosaic and less life-threatening issues you may notice as being quite common in bereaved clients is gastrointestinal (GI) problems. The sympathetic nervous system dominance over the parasympathetic nervous system, which often prevails when there is a fight-or-flight response, will frequently affect the digestive system adversely. For many, their digestive system may already tend to be reactive to stress during 'normal' times. Grief is obviously an extreme stressor, and if your client is already sensitive to GI disturbances, the stress of grief can mean these symptoms become even more problematic. Bereaved clients may complain of any of the usual digestive issues that you may be familiar with seeing, such as nausea, constipation, diarrhoea, bloating, flatulence, heartburn and acid reflux. Changes in appetite are also common, particularly in early grief, and your client may tell you about a sensation of feeling an emptiness or gnawing in the stomach. As well as obviously addressing these digestive issues just as you might normally do, extra reassurance that these symptoms can be common in grief is important, especially if these issues are unfamiliar to them. Using myself as an example, I don't usually experience digestive problems, but I found the unanticipated nausea and strange gnawing sensation in my stomach during early grief very disconcerting. These extra physical symptoms can sometimes feel overwhelming for grievers on top of the full-on emotional pain of their loss, so normalizing their occurrence and explaining that they are usually transitory and that you have suggestions that could help will be reassuring for the client.

STUDIES ON THE PHYSICAL SYMPTOMS OF GRIEF

There is a surprising amount of research into the effects of grief – studies that, for example, show that becoming widowed is associated with an increase in risk of mortality of between 48 and 66 per cent within the first few months of bereavement; that the likelihood of bereaved spouses having a sudden cardiac death rises significantly in the six months following a death; and that traumatic grief symptoms can precede illnesses such as cancer. Inflammation, already highlighted, plays a significant role.

One study, entitled 'Grief, depressive symptoms, and inflammation in the spousally bereaved', found the following:

> In the initial months after the loss of a spouse, those who are widowed are at risk for cardiovascular problems and premature mortality... Bereaved individuals with a higher grief severity had higher levels of the proinflammatory cytokines IFN-γ, IL-6, and TNF-α than those with less grief severity.[5]

This is the first study to demonstrate that, based on grief severity, inflammatory markers can distinguish that those widowed with a high grief severity had greater levels of inflammation compared with those whose grief is less severe.

In another study, 'History of sudden unexpected loss is associated with elevated interleukin-6 and decreased insulin-like growth factor-1 in women in an urban primary care setting',[6] the hypothesis that a history of sudden unexpected loss, including number of losses and type of loss (death due to unnatural versus natural causes), would be associated with the magnitude of dysregulation was investigated. They concluded that sudden unexpected death of a loved one confers risk of morbidity and mortality, probably due to dysregulation in the immune/inflammatory and endocrine systems.

Increased blood pressure, chest pain, irregular heartbeat and heart attacks are associated with the stress that grief can have on the cardiovascular system, so be aware that you could come across this in a bereaved client and will obviously need to refer them to their GP if necessary. However, it's really not unusual after a significant loss to feel physical pain in your heart, as well as a tightness in your chest

5   Fagundes *et al.*, 2019, p.190
6   Cankaya *et al.*, 2009

(again, I can personally vouch for this), and there are several studies to be found on broken heart syndrome, also known as reversible heart failure. This is now becoming recognized as a very real medical issue. It is found, almost exclusively, in post-menopausal women – so please watch out for this in that particular age group of bereaved women. Apparently, scans show that the heart of someone with broken heart syndrome can look identical to the heart of someone who has heart disease. Fortunately, however, broken heart syndrome can usually be reversed, given time.

The study 'Distinguishing a heart attack from the "broken heart syndrome" (Takotsubo cardiomyopathy)' states the following regarding broken heart syndrome:

> It may mimic an acute myocardial infarction, accompanied by minimal elevation of cardiac enzymes, usually without evidence of obstructive coronary artery disease. Most clinicians are unfamiliar with this disorder... Enhanced awareness by clinicians is important when encountering patients with chest pain and elevated cardiac enzymes. Takotsubo cardiomyopathy (broken heart syndrome) is usually associated with a favorable prognosis, although in rare instances it may be associated with life-threatening complications.[7]

It seems fairly conclusive, then, that grief has the ability to seriously affect our health, as well as potentially shorten life expectancy, particularly in widows/widowers and bereaved parents. One study published in *BMJ Supportive and Palliative Care* followed more than 1000 bereaved parents and found that parents in Scotland were more than twice as likely to die in the first 15 years following their child's death as parents who had not lost a child. Among bereaved mothers in England and Wales, the risk of early death was four times higher than non-bereaved parents. Mairi Harper, who led the study, says: 'There is evidence that bereavement is a risk factor for illness. We did

7   Nussinovitch *et al.*, 2011, p.524

expect that bereaved parents would show a higher illness factor, but we did not expect their risk to be as great as it was.'[8] The study suggests several reasons for the increased rates of death among bereaved parents, such as weakened immune systems or the probability of some long-lasting effects caused by the stress of their loss. However, the authors noted that lifestyle factors such as alcohol consumption, poor diet and general lack of self-care during grief may sometimes play a part, and they did not rule out suicide as a cause of death.

In November 2021, an article by Nicholas Bakalar in *The New York Times*, 'The loss of a child takes a physical toll on the heart',[9] highlighted new research looking at the damage done to the hearts of parents who lost children of all ages up until the age of 29. The risk of a heart attack for grieving parents in the first week after the loss of their child was assessed to be triple the rate of people who had not lost a child, and an increased risk can persist for years. Bakalar quotes Dr Erica Spatz, an associate professor of cardiovascular medicine at Yale: 'The loss of a child plays out in every aspect of a patient's life, including their cardiovascular health.' The article goes on to suggest that patients should be screened for this trauma among other factors. Child loss, the article says, 'is a very special type of bereavement, one of the greatest stresses that one can experience'. While it's difficult perhaps to deliver this information of a significantly increased cardiovascular risk to bereaved parents, Bakalar continues, 'it's important for doctors, friends and family members of a person who has lost a child to be on the lookout for things like chest pain, shortness of breath or other signs of heart problems or impending heart attack'. As wellness practitioners, it will be essential for us to also be aware of these risk factors if we find ourselves working with a bereaved parent.

Suicidal ideation can be prevalent among the bereaved, particularly if the death of the loved one was sudden, and even more so if the death was by suicide. Suicidal ideation is also very common among bereaved parents, regardless of the cause of death, and sometimes

8   Gann, 2011
9   Bakalar, 2021

bereaved siblings, too. Obviously, you will need to refer on if you have a client you believe to be in danger of taking their own life, but it is perhaps necessary to point out here that it is quite possible that these feelings can very much be part of the grieving process when someone finds themselves in a position where they just can't imagine living without their loved one and are suffering from the extraordinary shock and unbearable emotional pain that they perceive to be impossible to survive. Most, in time, get past these feelings, but it's important that they don't feel stigmatized for having them and are allowed be open about how they're feeling. Again, your compassion is paramount.

One study, 'Perceived stigma of sudden bereavement as a risk factor for suicidal thoughts and suicide attempt: Analysis of British cross-sectional survey data on 3387 young bereaved adults',[10] concluded:

> The sudden death of a friend or relative, particularly by suicide, is a risk factor for suicide. People who experience sudden bereavement report feeling highly stigmatised by the loss, potentially influencing access to support... Subjects with high perceived stigma scores were significantly more likely to report post-bereavement suicidal thoughts than those with low stigma scores. People who feel highly stigmatised by a sudden bereavement are at increased risk of suicidal thoughts and suicide attempt, even taking into account prior suicidal behaviour. General practitioners, bereavement counsellors, and others who support people bereaved suddenly, should consider inquiring about perceived stigma, mental wellbeing, and suicidal thoughts, and directing them to appropriate sources of support.

Although I believe it's very necessary to be aware of all of the above research, it's probably more likely you will be addressing grief-related physical symptoms such as insomnia, fatigue, anxiety and IBS. However, knowledge of the more serious ramifications of loss may

---

10 Pitman *et al.*, 2017

ensure that you enquire more deeply and would be able to uncover something potentially more serious, as well as now possessing a greater understanding of the enormous impact grief can have, both immediately after the event and further down the line. Being able to explain this to your client, putting the emphasis on how vital it is for them to take care of their health and wellbeing – and how you might support them in doing so – will be invaluable.

Many of you will be aware that emotions can get stuck in the body if not allowed expression, storing up problems for later. As grief is generally so badly dealt with in our society, this is yet another good reason to allow your grieving client to express how they feel during your consultations. You will also be able to help your client by explaining how important it is to avoid suppressing their grief in any way and by advising on ways to release it, not just through outlets such as talking and crying but through walking, yoga, creativity, journaling, getting out in nature, etc.

BRAIN FUNCTION IN GRIEF

Grief rearranges the brain, according to Megan Devine. Grief can result in memory loss, confusion, not being able to pay attention and brain fog – or, as Devine calls it in her book *It's OK That You're Not OK*,[11] 'grief brain'. This has the potential to affect someone both physically and mentally, and it can be quite frightening if you haven't anticipated it playing such a major factor in the grieving process. Be aware that this type of brain fog is not only due to insomnia; both trauma and grief can interfere with our ability to think clearly. This is because the body gets flooded with cortisol, which can lead to feelings of confusion, fogginess and lack of concentration.

It's known that emotional traumatic brain 'injury' following the death of a loved one can result in definitive changes to brain function. According to neurologist Lisa M. Shulman, when we think about brain trauma, we usually think about physical injury, but it is

---

11   Devine, 2017

now understood that the emotional trauma of loss has a profound effect on the mind, brain and body.

> As our understanding of physical traumatic brain injury has expanded to include concussive sports injury, it's time to expand the definition to include *emotional traumatic brain injury*. It wasn't so long ago, that concussions were considered harmless; athletes were routinely returned to the field after they appeared to recover from being dazed or unconscious. We now understand that although no injury is seen on MRI or CT scans of the brain, brain injury has occurred. In the same way, the emotional trauma of loss results in serious changes in brain function that endure. The brain kicks into action to protect us during traumatic experience. Imagine what would happen if we weren't able to function during traumatic times. To sustain function and survival, the brain acts as a filter sensing the threshold of emotions and memories that we can and cannot handle. So the brain is especially active in managing the stress of traumatic loss.[12]

Megan Devine suggests in her book[13] that you imagine you have 100 units of brain power for each day. Then imagine that around 99 of these energy units have now been taken up by grief, trauma, sadness, etc., which leaves just one unit for normal daily activities. This is a great way of explaining it to your bereaved client if they are experiencing grief-related brain fog. Knowing they're not alone in how they feel is so important. Grief can be a destabilizing experience, so 'normalizing' both their emotional and physical expressions of grief is vital and can relieve some of the anxiety they may be feeling.

We will look at trauma in more detail in Chapter 4, but a traumatized brain has to work extra hard and will generally be overactive. When there has been trauma, the brain can't discern whether something happened in the past or is actually happening in the present,

---

12   Shulman, 2018
13   Devine, 2017

and sometimes it will relive the trauma in flashbacks, recreating the traumatic event(s). A traumatized brain is always on high alert and works much harder than a non-traumatized brain to keep up with everyday situations. This is exhausting and somewhat terrifying, as you can imagine. In many cases, grief-related trauma is going to need to be specifically addressed, although you can reassure your grieving client that the brain fog is likely to improve and that this will most probably be dependent on the passing of time and getting past the initial shock of their loss. However, perhaps be aware that many bereaved people report living with it, albeit to a lesser degree, for some considerable length of time.

THE EFFECTS OF DEHYDRATION IN GRIEF

Most of you will advise your clients to drink plenty of water, regardless of what they come to see you for. This is especially important during grief as it's thought that you can become dehydrated from crying when the grief is especially intense. It's possible, too, that the physiological effects of grief could result in dehydration, even when there have been few tears and the sufferer is remembering to drink. Extreme stress can cause dehydration and dehydration can cause an excessive release of cortisol. It can potentially exacerbate brain fog, not to mention grief-related stress, anxiety and depression. Under a microscope, tears of grief are shown to have a different chemical makeup to other kinds of tears. It's thought that emotional tears contain stress hormones, which the body releases in the process of crying. While highlighting the importance of drinking enough water when grieving, it might also be prudent to emphasize that tears are healing and so should never be suppressed.

COMPLIANCE AND YOUR GRIEVING CLIENT

If you're a nutritional therapist, you will be able to advise on supplements to support the brain and nervous system, as well as dietary measures, but every wellness practitioner can advise on sleep (so important for processing the emotional pain, yet sometimes so cruelly elusive during grief) and gentle exercise, plus any other suggestions you feel qualified to give, depending on what you practise.

However, please remember that with this current 'brain impairment', your suggestions may not be fully taken in, so it's a good idea to get your client to write everything down. Nevertheless, even if they do this, compliance may not be as great as you might hope, simply because they are coping with so much physically and emotionally, and are likely to feel completely exhausted and overwhelmed by it all. The effort of getting a meal on the table may well feel impossible initially, so please just go with this and meet them with understanding and compassion.

Even though I'm a nutritional therapist and fully understood the importance of good nutrition, I couldn't eat anything at all when first bereaved, and then for several weeks relied entirely on kind friends bringing meals (invariably a pasta bake and a crumble) or ordering takeaways. I did take my supplements, though, and you could put this to your client as an 'insurance policy' if they have no appetite or feel unable to shop or cook initially. By all means explain to them that they may feel better if they try to eat regular meals, always with protein, as their blood sugar balance may have been negatively affected by the extreme stress they've been under, but wait a little before sensitively explaining how the stress of grief and trauma can increase inflammation, affect the immune system, compromise digestion and deplete energy levels, and that the better their diet is, the stronger they will be physically. They may not care about any of this when they're in the initial pain of their loss and their life suddenly looks so different, but there will be a time when they're ready to hear it and then you can properly get to work. Those of you who provide more 'hands-on' treatments are very much needed during the initial stages of grief and can provide so much in the way of gentle healing for a wounded soul.

WEIGHT FLUCTUATIONS IN GRIEF

If you're a nutritional therapist, you may find a client comes to you for either weight gain or weight loss that has become an issue since their bereavement. It's quite usual with shock and trauma that there can be a loss of appetite and consequently weight loss, which is sometimes quite rapid. This should start to balance out in a few weeks, but obviously it is important to be alert to a past history of an eating disorder which may have been re-triggered by grief. Grief is a time when people feel they have no control over what's happened to them, and although, as we know, it's a complex issue, control can frequently play a part in eating disorders such as anorexia. Grief therefore can unfortunately provide the perfect conditions for a worsening, or resurgence, of this. It goes without saying that, whatever type of wellness practitioner you are, if you suspect anorexia in your client, you will need to refer them to their GP or to an eating disorder specialist if you know of one.

Weight gain through comfort eating is very common, usually developing a few weeks or months after the loss. An extra layer of padding may symbolize protection from the emotional hurt that is being endured. From a physiological perspective, an increase in cortisol caused by stress can contribute to cravings and weight gain. So, as we might expect, most weight issues under these circumstances are usually stemming from the pain of grief and may well right themselves as the client gets more accustomed to their new situation. As they do so, they may gradually begin to care more about re-establishing a healthier diet and lifestyle. A desire to do something about their weight gain can be seen as a positive sign of self-care and being ready to move forward in their grieving journey, although in some cases this may not happen for months or even years. And even if they do start to make progress, don't be surprised if their grief – particularly around anniversaries, birthdays and holidays – throws them off course. You may see a fair bit of 'two steps forward, one back', more so than with your non-grieving clients. Grief can knock your self-esteem, as already mentioned, so gentle encouragement for self-compassion if they fall off the wagon will go a long way.

DIET, SUPPLEMENTS, HERBS, HOMEOPATHIC REMEDIES, FLOWER ESSENCES

If you're a nutritional therapist, naturopath or herbalist, you will have plenty to offer your grieving client in terms of dietary advice, supplements and herbs to support their overall health during the grieving process, and I will expand on this in Chapter 9. However, it's important to remember that some clients may have visited their GP prior to coming to you and may well have been put on a (most probably very long) waiting list for bereavement counselling and, in the meantime, come away with a prescription for antidepressants or sleeping medication. This can be frustrating if you have some good supplement or herbal protocols for dealing with sleep, low mood, anxiety, etc., only to find these are contraindicated with their medication. Nevertheless, there will be much you can do using diet and lifestyle, and you may have other areas you can focus on supplement-wise (provided there are no contraindications), such as reducing inflammation, supporting the nervous and digestive systems, etc.

If you're a homeopath or you use flower essences in your clinic, you will also have some fantastic remedies to support a grieving client. Homeopathic remedies for grief include Ignatia, and my understanding is that it is one of the first remedies to consider after a significant loss or when grief is prolonged. Aconite can be helpful for shock. Of course, a consultation with a homeopath will ensure that the client is treated as an individual with a unique set of concerns and different miasms, and therefore there may be other remedies that are more appropriate than these. Flower remedies can offer some immediate relief, especially Rescue Remedy and also Star of Bethlehem, which can assist with the distress following a shock.

TESTING

With certain clients, tests can be useful for identifying an underlying root cause of dysfunction. If you're a nutritional therapist, you may use tests to establish if there are specific issues with, for example, the thyroid, adrenals, gut health or nutritional deficiencies. You may think it could be helpful to establish whether any of the above are a possibility with your grieving client. However, perhaps bear in mind that many tests involve reading instructions, collecting samples at very specific times, keeping them at a certain temperature until ready to send, arranging collection, etc., which may all be a bit too much for someone in early grief who is fatigued and possibly suffering from brain fog. In any case, testing when symptoms have only appeared since the loss may not be necessary when the underlying cause is likely to be grief and therefore the symptoms could well dissipate naturally given time and with your comprehensive support. If they don't, then testing could be an option further down the line.

OTHER RECOMMENDATIONS YOU CAN SHARE WITH YOUR CLIENT

It's quite likely that your client understands that they need to eat well, exercise and get enough sleep, but sometimes either this will not be possible for them in their current state or, bearing in mind the emotional impact of their loss, it may not feel like a priority for them. Just getting through the day may be enough of a challenge. Tactful encouragement to eat simple healthy meals, take gentle exercise and develop a good bedtime routine is all you can do if this is the case – and, above all, offer compassion for their immensely challenging situation.

Eventually, they may be more ready to take small proactive steps, and getting outside may be one of the best starting points. There is plenty of evidence to suggest that walking and being in nature can help with anxiety and emotional wellbeing. Nature really does heal, according to Louise Delagran at the University of Minnesota. Being in nature reduces anger, fear and stress, all of which may be experienced during grief.

Exposure to nature not only makes you feel better emotionally, it contributes to your physical wellbeing, reducing blood pressure, heart rate, muscle tension, and the production of stress hormones… In one study in *Mind*, 95% of those interviewed said their mood improved after spending time outside, changing from depressed, stressed, and anxious to more calm and balanced.[14]

Anecdotally, my grief coaching clients, my bereaved parents' group and, last but not least, I myself find that walking and being outside in nature is significant in easing some of the heaviness of grief.

We know that exercise is useful for expending the body's stress hormones, adrenaline and cortisol, which, if excessive, can be problematic during and after a trauma. Studies including 'Regular exercise is associated with emotional resilience to acute stress in healthy adults'[15] show that exercise may lower some of the negative health effects associated with stress, such as high cortisol. Exercise also increases the levels of endorphins, the body's natural painkillers and mood boosters. Walking is particularly good for grievers because it combines exercise with being out in nature with all its benefits. To literally put one foot in front of the other, to take one step at a time, symbolizes the emotional effort we sometimes have to make to get through each day when we're on an often unforgiving journey of grief. They say it's important to look up and out, as it helps to remember the vastness of the sky when your world has shrunk, and this also makes both walking and nature incredibly important to healing when someone is grieving.

Yoga is a form of exercise of particular benefit during grief, and you could recommend an online yoga class such as Yoga with Adriene.[16] – I love her 'yoga for grief'. The simple breathing and stretching exercises can be invaluable for calming anxiety, and because yoga combines movement with breathing, it can lead to a positive physiological and emotional response, calming an over-triggered nervous

---

14 Delagran, n.d.
15 Childs and de Wit, 2014
16 https://yogawithadriene.com

system and promoting relaxation. This has been shown to help with symptoms of PTSD, so often experienced when the loss has been traumatic (see Chapter 4).

If you have a grieving client, it is quite likely that they may have problems with sleep. Not being able to sleep when you're grieving can feel like torture. You can go to dark places when the rest of the world is asleep, not to mention getting unpleasant adrenaline rushes when you wake up suddenly during the night. Supplements or herbs can help to a certain extent, if you're qualified to offer them and your client doesn't have any medication contraindications. If the latter is the case, or supplements and herbs aren't your area of expertise, then you can make other suggestions. You will probably have your own recommendations, but finding a sleep meditation or using a breathing technique would be something you might offer. One of the simplest techniques is to count slowly back from 100, repeating until you fall asleep.

You could also suggest the 4-7-8 technique (breathe in for a count of 4, hold for a count of 7 and breathe out slowly through the mouth for 8), both to help with insomnia and also for any time of day or night when they feel anxious. It is thought that the lengthening of the exhale helps to soothe an agitated nervous system and that this simple action can halt the flood of stress hormones that can trigger an escalation of anxiety.

However, please note that something like a breathing technique – while totally valid in theory – can sound a somewhat trite suggestion coming from someone who isn't going through what they're going through. I know addressing my breathing really helps my grief-related anxiety and insomnia, but sometimes, when you're going through the dark night of the soul, it can be impossible to implement even the simplest of suggestions.

CHAPTER 4

Mental Health, Trauma and PTSD

You may feel that mental health is not your area of expertise. Most wellness practitioners aren't psychologists or psychotherapists and probably don't hold a qualification in mental health. However, it's useful for all of us to have some understanding of how grief impacts our mental health, as well as how useful it is as a practitioner to become 'trauma-informed'. This will be helpful not just for your grieving client but for many of your other clients, too. You may already have some knowledge of ACEs – adverse childhood experiences. If so, you will know the major impact that trauma of any kind, in childhood or more recently, has on our health and wellbeing. There are now many continuing professional development (CPD) courses available to assist you in becoming trauma-informed, and you may find, with awareness around trauma definitely on the rise, that more and more clients will start seeking a trauma-informed practitioner. We have already looked at some of the issues caused by grief in Chapter 3, but now we will go into further detail about how grief and trauma can affect your client's mental health, including how common PTSD is with certain types of loss, such as sudden death, finding a loved one dead, witnessing a death, loss of a child and cumulative losses.

The controversial 'prolonged grief' criteria aside, grief in itself isn't a mental health issue, but grief can involve anxiety and depression, both of which are. It may be that your client has no prior history of anxiety or depression, or it may be that they do, and grief has exacerbated the severity of these issues. Grief and trauma can potentially re-trigger past issues your client had thought they had worked through and resolved, such as self-harming, addiction or an eating disorder. Equally, if the loss was very traumatic, these issues can appear for the first time. It's a good idea to enquire sensitively about the possibility of any of these serious mental health disorders and then recommend they seek some specialist help, as these issues will be outside the remit of most wellness practitioners. Regarding anxiety and mild to moderate depression in grief, if you have tools or protocols that you would normally use to support somebody experiencing these issues, then use them, but refer on if you don't feel confident in doing so or it proves not to be enough. (See Chapter 9 for what might help in terms of nutritional medicine.)

People who experience trauma and loss are confronted with a new version of themselves that they have no choice in, and this can be destabilizing, scary and very overwhelming. Some will do their best to adjust to this new version of themselves, but others will struggle to do so and may seek help. Although typically it's all that's offered, traditional talk-based approaches are unlikely to be enough, or indeed appropriate, where traumatic grief is concerned. (See the section on PTSD below for further expansion on this.) Traumatic loss may call for less traditional interventions. These include body-based therapies, energy healing, somatic body work and spiritual/intuitive practices to address the spirit/soul aspects of death. It may be useful to pass this on to a client who may be confused as to why talk-based therapy or counselling hasn't left them feeling any better. I've heard many times that bereavement counselling or therapy hasn't 'worked' when there is trauma involved in grief.

It may empower your client if you can reinforce that they are the true expert in their grief journey and may intuitively know what – and who – is best placed to help them. Unfortunately, trauma can sometimes override that intuition, so encouragement to trust it again (which can be challenging in a world that now feels unsafe) may help with their healing. As a practitioner, you can also use your own intuition to think outside the box about how best to support your client's needs – you may not personally have the complete skill set necessary, but you can point them in the right direction, referring them to a book, a specialist practitioner or an online resource. Above all, think holistically about your client's grief experience from the perspective of mind, body and spirit.

OLD WOUNDS

Aside from the emotional upheaval commonly associated with the grieving process, grief can also bring to the surface the additional pain of old wounds. This is because grief has a tendency to trigger the parts of us that are unhealed. These wounds often stem from childhood, though not always. If viewed with a positive slant, the re-emergence of these old wounds provides an opportunity for them to be finally healed. Our capacity for healing will depend here on our willingness to fully feel *all* of our painful feelings, regardless of where they stem from. We can't heal what we don't feel, as they say, and sometimes, if we're to move forward, it's going to be necessary to get comfortable with feeling uncomfortable while we process everything, including wounds from the past that may not have been fully dealt with at the time. You may decide this is beyond your scope as a wellness practitioner. However, you can still help your client to make sense of what's happening, explaining that it's common for grief to act as a trigger for these buried feelings. This is especially true if they have an abandonment wound because it's not unusual to feel 'abandoned' by the person who has died. That feeling might then bring up memories of when they felt like this before.

THE STRESS OF GRIEF

You will probably be very used to seeing clients who experience stress, and some of them may specifically seek your expertise for dealing with it. Stress is considered to be anything that has the potential to upset our equilibrium. Stress is obviously not always traumatic, but traumatic experiences are always stressful. When someone experiences a traumatic event, their body's defences take effect and create a stress response.

According to PsychCentral, the first phase, or the 'alarm reaction', occurs immediately on contact with a stressor, such as at the death of a loved one:

> At the death the brain 'translates' the stress of grief into a chemical reaction in the body. The pituitary gland located at the base of the brain is stimulated to produce a hormone called adrenocorticotrophin hormone (ACTH). This reaction is a 'protective' one and in essence makes the body ready to do battle. The ACTH (from the pituitary gland) then travels to the adrenal gland, a gland at the top of the kidneys, which causes a chemical reaction which ultimately produces cortisone. As the cortisone level increases it causes the production of ACTH to level off. What happens in the case of grief where the stress continues for many months? The cycle does not operate as it should. Because the stress is continuing, the production of ACTH is continuing thus causing the adrenal gland to produce more and more cortisone. The result is an abnormally high level of cortisone circulating in the blood sometimes exceeding ten to twenty times the normal levels.[1]

This description of the chemistry involved when we come up against an extreme stressor, such as the death of a loved one, leads, as discussed in Chapter 3, to an increased susceptibility to illness, changes in eating habits, problems with sleep, brain fog, etc. And, as discussed in the section on secondary losses in Chapter 1, there will then be other stressors to cope with in addition to the loss itself, stacking up the amount of emotional and physical stressors that your client has to deal with. According to PsychCentral:

---

1   Gray, 2016

The majority of bereaved people experience some kind of physical illness in the first four to six months after the death of their loved one. For most the illness can be directly tied into the extreme stress of their loved one's death... [I]f you have damaged your body in the early months of grief you run the risk of never completely recovering from the physical illness – and recovery for bereaved people means recovery in body as well as mind.[2]

DEPRESSION IN YOUR GRIEVING CLIENT

Depression is likely to play some part in the grieving process and is one stage of Elisabeth Kübler-Ross's well-known five stages of grief: denial, anger, bargaining, depression and acceptance. (The merits of this grief model are now being challenged, which will be explored further in Chapter 7.) It is, for instance, normal to feel enormous sadness and want to withdraw for a while in order to process the loss. One of the important differences between clinical depression and the depression that's often experienced as a natural part of the grieving process is that, in grief, the depression is more likely to fluctuate and come in waves. Often, the depression seen during the grieving process will eventually pass, but in some cases it won't.

We have already looked at complicated grief in Chapter 1 – found commonly in a bereaved person when their loved one has died before their time, and/or suddenly and unexpectedly, and/or through suicide or murder – and it is here that depression is found to be most prevalent and persistent. This kind of grief can be all-consuming and overwhelming, and there may be a feeling of hopelessness, lack of self-worth and suicidal ideation. If you have sufficient trust and rapport, your client may share these feelings with you, and it's possible that they may not have done so with anyone else. (It can be a lot for those around them to take on the weight of their grief and trauma, and the client may not want to burden them – and not all

---

2   Ibid.

grievers have counsellors.) This can feel like quite a responsibility for a wellness practitioner.

Although you will be bound to refer them to their GP if you're concerned about them being a danger to themselves, you can explain to them that the level of depression they feel is hardly surprising considering the trauma they have experienced. Once again, your compassion will be paramount. Signs of depression in grief that you can look out for might include long-term trouble sleeping, poor appetite beyond the first few weeks, fatigue, difficulty in getting out of bed and excessive and frequent crying spells. There may also be feelings of loneliness, isolation, emptiness and anxiety. Although most wellness practitioners need to tread very carefully and refer on when the depression is deep and long-term, there are still some ways you can support your client, as we will see later in this chapter and also in Chapters 9 and 10.

ANXIETY IN YOUR GRIEVING CLIENT

When you've lost someone, it's very common to fear losing someone else – it's happened once, so it might happen again. You need to be alert and prepared for the next terrible event that might happen. Anxiety is a normal and necessary basic human emotion designed to keep us safe, but when there is no threat immediately present or the anxiety is disproportionate to a threat, then anxiety is considered problematic and a potential mental health issue. As previously mentioned, living through traumatic loss means that the world now feels like a very unsafe one, a place where very bad things can happen – and you now have concrete evidence of this. It is probably fair to say that if your grieving client suffered from anxiety or an anxiety disorder before their bereavement, they may well find that this is exacerbated by grief. This may diminish given time and through implementation of the breathing techniques outlined in Chapter 3, as well as diet and supplements (see Chapter 9), the various alternative therapies outlined below, and the advice to be found in Chapter 10.

Studies indicate that diet quality is generally poorer in those with depressive and anxiety disorders,[3] and that's without factoring the other issues that can be commonly found with grief. However, we will now move on to an extreme form of anxiety sometimes present with traumatic loss – PTSD – which is classed as an anxiety disorder.

PTSD IN GRIEF

So, what's the difference between experiencing a trauma and going on to develop PTSD? Trauma is an actual event. It can be any event that causes psychological, physical, emotional or mental harm, including a death. The main difference is that a traumatic event is time-based, whereas PTSD is a longer-term condition where someone continues to have flashbacks, re-experiences the traumatic event and has associated ongoing physical or mental symptoms. Hypervigilance (an elevated state of constantly being over alert to potential threats around you) and increased arousal (living in a state of constant tension or feeling wired, affecting the ability to relax or sleep) are two of the hallmarks of PTSD.

According to PTSD UK,[4] it's estimated that 50 per cent of people will experience a trauma at some point in their life, and although the majority of people exposed to traumatic events only experience some short-term distress, around 20 per cent of people who experience a trauma go on to develop PTSD (so around one in ten people at some point in their lives).

PTSD is essentially a memory filing error caused by a traumatic event. When you experience something really traumatic your body suspends 'normal operations' and so temporarily shuts down some bodily functions such as digestion, skin repair and crucially, memory processing. During trauma, your brain thinks 'processing and

---

3   Gibson-Smith *et al.*, 2018
4   PTSD UK, n.d.(a)

understanding what is going on right now is not important! Getting your legs ready to run, your heart rate up, and your arms ready to fight this danger is what's important right now. I'll get back to the processing later.' As such, until the danger passes, the mind does not produce a memory for this traumatic event in the normal way. So, when your brain eventually does go back to try to process the trauma, and the mind presents the situation as a memory for filing, it finds it 'does not exist' in your memory yet, so it sees it as a situation in the current timeline, and so it can be very distressing. The distress comes from the fact that the brain is unable to recognise this as a 'memory', because it hasn't been processed as one. As such, the facts of what happened, the emotions associated with the trauma and the sensations touch, taste, sound, vision, movement, and smell can be presented by the mind in the form of flashbacks – as if they are happening right now. The distress during the traumatic event, and this continued distress is what causes that change in the brain, and the subsequent symptoms of PTSD.

It's not clear why some people develop PTSD, while others who've been in a similar situation don't develop the condition. Interestingly, however, women have a two to three times higher risk of developing PTSD compared with men. According to PTSD UK, the lifetime prevalence of PTSD is about 10–12 per cent in women and 5–6 per cent in men. Women also appear to have a more sensitized hypothalamus–pituitary axis than men, which could perhaps explain the prevalence.[5]

It's possible that, given time, PTSD symptoms will dissipate naturally, but often they won't. In that case, if you suspect your client has PTSD (and not everyone gets a diagnosis or realizes they might have it), you will need to suggest that they find appropriate and effective support, the nature of which can vary from person to person and which might be beyond your scope. As a nutritional therapist, I do

---

5   Ibid.

believe there are dietary measures and personalized supplement protocols that can, in part, help and which I outline in Chapter 9, but as someone who has personal experience of PTSD, I consider it to be a very complex condition, and it may inevitably benefit from a combination of approaches. Don't expect to have all the answers.

My own experience of seeking alternative therapies that might help with PTSD is that some wellness practitioners are convinced their particular modality will solve everything for you (especially if they have perhaps had some success with clients who have issues stemming from childhood trauma as opposed to a more recent traumatic loss). In fact, they are out of their depth with such a serious and distressing disorder, and I feel very strongly that PTSD needs to be addressed very responsibly and not by those without training and experience in this area, or at the very least only by those who have done some extensive research into the condition. It is hoped, though, that this book can begin to make us all better informed on the complexity of PTSD, even if we decide to refer on.

It's a truly horrible and debilitating condition, and something no one would wish on their worst enemy. Those of us who have PTSD can very easily find ourselves reliving the traumatic event where the intense fear and pain first became embedded. It's incredibly scary to live with this condition, where any small trigger can lead to horrifying flashbacks or full-on fight, flight or freeze. It's commonly assumed that PTSD is just about the flashbacks, but any stressor can trigger the physical symptoms of being on high alert – the body remembers the imprint of the traumatic event and 'keeps the score'. We may understand intellectually why we have this response, but to energetically release these emotions from the body is often easier said than done.

My personal observation, through my work as a 'trauma-informed' holistic grief coach, is that nearly all bereaved parents I've worked with have PTSD to a greater or lesser degree (some have been given the diagnosis, some haven't), as do some of the widows/widowers, and young adults who have lost a parent or sibling, especially when the death was sudden. I listen and help them work through the grieving process, provide dietary and supplement advice on calming the nervous system and supporting the adrenals, get them to do breathing techniques, some havening (see below), and any other ideas or techniques I feel might support them. But I then often advise on how they might find additional help – even though I consider myself to be trauma-informed. It's not a condition you can just 'get over', and someone with PTSD may find it impossible to achieve sustainable recovery without specific treatment, and even then – and this is really important – it's by no means guaranteed. It's crucial, speaking from personal as well as professional experience, that as a wellness practitioner, of any kind, we don't ever claim to treat such a serious and complicated mental health issue, unless we are properly proficient.

SIGNS OF PTSD

Psychological

- Reliving the trauma through a distressing recall of the event, flashbacks, and nightmares.
- Constantly thinking about the traumatic event.
- Being easily irritated and angered.
- Emotional numbness.
- Detachment.
- Disorientation.
- Feeling unreal.
- Overwhelm.
- Fear.

Physical

- Increased arousal and anxiety, feelings of being on high alert.
- Disrupted sleep.
- Inability to concentrate.
- Nausea.
- Sweating.
- Racing heart.
- Trembling.
- Pain.

Social

- Avoiding places and people that might remind you of the trauma (even ones that don't directly do so can still provoke anxiety).
- Becoming isolated and withdrawn.
- Giving up activities you once enjoyed.
- Loss of purpose.

THE SCIENCE AND BIOLOGY OF PTSD

The reason for providing quite a lot of information on PTSD is because it's not always fully understood, particularly in the context of traumatic grief, and you may well see a grieving client who hasn't been formally diagnosed – in which case you will be able to raise with them the possibility that they may have it, enabling them to potentially seek the right help. The knowledge and awareness you will gain from this chapter could be useful to draw on.

The extreme stress resulting from PTSD can lead to both acute and chronic changes in neurochemical systems and specific brain regions, which result in long-term changes in the brain circuits. This mainly revolves around hormonal signals and the amygdala, hippocampus and medial prefrontal cortex within the brain. Here's a little detail on the parts of the brain that are involved in PTSD, as outlined by PTSD UK.

Amygdala

The amygdala is the part of the brain that formulates a response to stress. It takes this 'alert' from sensory input and, in response to per-ceived danger, sends out an 'alarm' to warn the rest of your body that various psychological actions are needed, such as activating fight, flight or freeze. When the danger or perceived danger has passed, new signals are transmitted to calm everything back down. In cases of PTSD, the amygdala is too sensitive, easily triggered, or remains on high alert for longer than it should. This results in hypervigilance and an extreme reaction to perceived threats. Having an overactive amygdala can lead to high levels of anxiety and poor sleep – this is something you may be able to help with, at least to some extent.[6]

---

6   Based on 'The science and biology of PTSD: Amygdala' in PTSD UK, n.d.(a)

Hippocampus

This part of the brain works together with the amygdala. The hippo-campus is where we store memories, and also the brain tissue that sorts and retrieves memories. PTSD can make this link 'unstable'. Someone who has experienced trauma may find, for example, that a loud noise sends them into a state of fear, possibly leading to flash-backs linking to their trauma. In this situation, the hippocampus does not supply the amygdala with the message to calm everything down.[7]

Medial prefrontal cortex

The prefrontal cortex deals with emotions and impulses, and there-fore has a substantial role to play in our actions. Usually, it would act in conjunction with your hippocampus, sending signals to your amygdala to switch off the alarm system when a situation calms down. With PTSD, this part of the brain is often underactive and 'dampened down' by the trauma. It's an involuntary defence mech-anism, creating emotional numbness so the trauma doesn't have to be relived. Low activity in the prefrontal cortex means it doesn't interact efficiently with your hippocampus and its store of memo-ries, and interferes with your amygdala alarm system's 'off switch'. Alternatively, a malfunctioning medial prefrontal cortex could make fear the dominant emotion. This also keeps your amygdala on high alert. Importantly, the frontal lobe is the part of the brain that deals with language skills. PTSD brain injury can therefore result in the individual struggling to articulate their emotions and thoughts.[8]

---

7   Based on 'The science and biology of PTSD: Hippocampus' in PTSD UK, n.d.(a).

8   Based on 'The science and biology of PTSD: Medial prefrontal cortex' in PTSD UK, n.d.(a)

'Deranged' cortisol levels

Cortisol is a stress warning to your body, and therefore it heightens alertness and creates fear. When your brain puts your body on full alert, the amount of cortisol produced increases. As we know, this can shut down other systems in the body in order to be ready for fight or flight. When the perceived danger is gone, your brain adjusts the production of cortisol, calming it down and so allowing the rest of your body to 'reset' back to normal. However, in PTSD this reset doesn't happen and you remain on high alert, impacting digestion and sleep. Elevated cortisol can result in issues with mood, concentration, migraines, depression and even heart attacks. However, not everyone with PTSD has too much cortisol; some have low levels instead.[9]

WHAT MIGHT HELP YOUR GRIEVING CLIENT WITH PTSD

Many traumatized people find themselves chronically out of sync with those around them, and so you may look like a lifeline for them. Their expectations of how you might help could be high, and you may therefore need to manage this. Although what has happened cannot ever be undone, it is possible for the imprints of trauma upon the mind, body and spirit to be effectively addressed, even though it's not always easy to get the right help. It can sometimes be a case of 'horses for courses'. For change to take place, the body needs to learn that the danger has passed and to live in the reality of the present, says Bessel Van Der Kolk.[10] A lot of treatment for PTSD looks at rewiring the connection between memories, emotions and behaviours, giving new associations and coping strategies, dismantling negative cycles and creating healthier brain function. Given that everyone is different, so too will the brain alterations, and emotional and behavioural responses of each individual be different. In the UK, the two main

---

9   Based on 'The science and biology of PTSD: "Deranged" cortisol levels' in PTSD UK, n.d.(a)
10   Van Der Kolk, 2014

psychological treatments conventionally recommended for treating PTSD are eye movement desensitization and reprocessing (EMDR) and cognitive behavioural therapy (CBT). Your client may be aware of these therapies or may seek your opinion on them, so here is a little information about them.

Eye movement desensitization and reprocessing (EMDR)

EMDR is a form of psychotherapy which is rapidly gaining credibility for treating PTSD. The fact that it doesn't rely on talking or medication may make it particularly appropriate for some. It can help eliminate the emotional aspects tied to memories of traumatic events by altering the manner in which the brain processes memories and other information. A 2014 review of scientific findings showed that as many as 90 per cent of trauma survivors overcame symptoms after just three EMDR sessions.[11] EMDR can produce measurable structural changes in the brain regions that are associated with fear conditioning. Another review of its efficacy in the treatment of PTSD concluded that overall 'EMDR is a useful, evidence-based tool for the treatment of post-traumatic stress disorder.'[12] However, according to a psychologist I spoke to, it should be noted that there is no guarantee it will work for everyone with PTSD that stems from traumatic loss and it may certainly take a much greater number of sessions than three. Your client can be referred for EMDR via their GP.

Cognitive behavioural therapy (CBT)

CBT is the other therapy that is commonly suggested for PTSD. One of the reasons it is offered to people with PTSD is that it can help them break down all their symptoms and difficulties into small,

---

11 Shapiro, 2014
12 Navarro *et al.*, 2018, p. 101

achievable goals, but CBT is not a quick fix, and it can take anything from a few weeks to six months to show substantial results. Also, some studies show that 'nonresponse' to CBT can be as high as 50 per cent, although this depends on various factors, including comorbidity and the nature of the populations studied.[13] According to PTSD UK,[14] for some people, negative and unhelpful connections between thoughts, emotions and behaviours can come back or manifest in new ways. It can also be difficult for people to engage with if they are feeling severely depressed or anxious (which is quite likely in cases of traumatic loss), not least because it relies on the individual creating their own coping strategies and new connections between thoughts and actions. This is obviously not easy to do when you are in a state of emotional over-arousal. In fact, a skilled therapist would need to be aware of when exploring a situation in CBT is increasing anxiety and depression, rather than achieving positive adjustments.

There are, however, many other therapies and activities that can be used to ease PTSD symptoms, whether your client is on a long waiting list for EMDR or CBT or you want to suggest something as a way of working alongside those treatments and your own modality. Some may have short-term effects, and some have long-term effects, but by having knowledge of what might potentially help, alongside your own method of support, they can be combined to provide a welcome source of possible relief for the draining, soul-sapping symptoms of PTSD.

Some of these therapies do not rely on the retelling of your story but rather address the physical implications in the present moment. This is perhaps one of the main differences between treating trauma and treating grief, and it should be emphasized that when addressing grief alone, the importance of the telling and retelling of the bereavement story is considered key to moving through grief. However, when talk therapy won't on its own shift complicated or traumatic

---

13   Kar, 2011
14   PTSD UK, n.d.(b)

grief, you might want to suggest physiological approaches such as body-based therapies and the creative arts (see Chapter 10).

Trauma comes back as a reaction, not a memory. One of the best books on trauma and PTSD, and how our bodies carry our experiences of traumatic events, is *The Body Keeps the Score* by Bessel Van Der Kolk.[15] Van Der Kolk says that the essence of trauma is that it is overwhelming, unbelievable and unbearable, and that it robs you of the feeling that you are in charge of yourself. He also says: 'As long as the trauma is not resolved, the stress hormones that the body secretes to protect itself keep circulating...and the emotional responses keep getting replayed.'[16] And this brings us back to why talking therapies alone may have limited efficacy in cases of PTSD due to its physical as well as emotional/mental expression. In fact, Van Der Kolk notes that 9/11 trauma survivors reported that acupuncture, massage, yoga and EMDR were what helped them the most, rather than the usual recommendations of traditional talk therapies made by so-called experts.

When someone has PTSD, there is a horrible feeling of being 'stuck', and we know this is because the neural pathways in the brain keep on perceiving danger when there isn't any. The more ingrained these neural pathways become, the more we are likely to repeat our reaction to a perceived threat. As I wrote in my book *Love Untethered*:

> Repetitive thoughts make the grooves deeper, contributing to our suffering, as can repeatedly telling your story. It's a fine balance because we do initially need to tell our story many times, whether to friends or a counsellor/therapist. However, in the long term, this may not be entirely helpful if we want to heal and create new neural pathways. Being in survival mode is meant to be a temporary phase that can help to save your life. It's not meant to be how you live once the immediate danger has passed. Unfortunately, sometimes when we

---

15   Van Der Kolk, 2014
16   Van Der Kolk, 2014, p.36

endure experiences that wound us so deeply, survival systems remain active. These systems shift us onto a different unfamiliar path, one we wouldn't be on if we hadn't been so disruptively traumatised.[17]

WHAT WE AS WELLNESS PRACTITIONERS CAN OFFER SOMEONE WITH PTSD

Although it might seem disheartening to your client that trauma has changed the way their brain functions, remind them that healing can change the way their brain functions, too. There is always hope, but equally it is always important to acknowledge that, for someone who is traumatized, it takes huge courage – more than you may be able to imagine – to attempt to heal after something terrible has happened. As wellness practitioners, most of us offer something that supports the wellbeing of the physical body. So, with all of the above in mind, many of us will have something to contribute to a grieving client with PTSD, even though it may need to be used in conjunction with another therapy. It will help to be aware that some of the physical complaints you might see, such as migraines and asthma, may, according to Van Der Kolk, be trauma responses in those supressing their trauma. Nutritional therapy applications can be found in Chapter 9, but here are a few other therapies that may help and, whether you practise any of them or not, you can suggest them to your client where you feel it's appropriate.

Acupuncture

In view of what Bessel Van Der Kolk has to say about 9/11 trauma survivors finding acupuncture more helpful than talk-based therapy, this is most definitely worth suggesting to your client. If you're an acupuncturist yourself, then you could potentially make a huge difference to those with PTSD. Acupuncture can act on parts of the brain known

---

17   May, 2022, p.141

for reducing sensitivity to stress and helps promote relaxation as well as combatting other issues such as lack of energy and disrupted sleep. According to the research, acupuncture can affect the autonomic nervous system, and the prefrontal as well as limbic brain structures, which is what makes it able to relieve the symptoms of PTSD effectively.[18]

Reiki

There are numerous studies to be found citing reiki as a potentially effective treatment for anxiety and depression. It definitely helped me, particularly in the early stages of grief. I felt reiki soothed my soul as well as my nervous system and helped me sleep better, and I just felt a little more able to cope with my grief and trauma after a session. According to an article about reiki and PTSD:

> Reiki, simply stated, calms and stills the spirit of the person. It can promote relaxation from the outside in and remind the body how it feels to be calm again... Oftentimes, emotions can get trapped and stored in the body as cellular memory. Through deep relaxation and calming of the spirit, those trapped or buried emotions and trauma can be gently released. It is important to remember that Reiki heals at the soul or spirit level, thus we can never predict the person's experience or outcome. Trusting and following the energy will always take us where we need to go and address what the person needs most in that moment... [T]he most important thing to know when giving Reiki is that it acts on priority. This means that it gives the person what they most need at that moment in time...not what we think they need... Let the person and his energy guide you and show you what he needs.[19]

I particularly like that this method of healing is spirit- or soul-based

18 Ding *et al.*, 2020
19 Lipinski, 2012

and not just focused on the involvement of body and brain. This very much ties in with my experience that grief and trauma involve the mind, body and spirit.

Emotional freedom technique (EFT)

Some of you may practise EFT, but if you're unfamiliar with it, EFT stands for emotional freedom technique and is sometimes called 'psychological acupressure' or tapping. It's a scientifically proven technique that works to rewire the brain by sending calming signals to the amygdala, the stress centre of the brain, allowing both the body and brain to release emotional blockages. These techniques are being accepted increasingly in medical and psychiatric circles as well as in the range of psychotherapies and healing disciplines. EFT is considered beneficial for trauma, anxiety and depression. The treatment involves the use of fingertips to tap on the end points of energy meridians situated just beneath the surface of the skin while focusing on an emotional trigger in order to release it.

EFT is a simple-to-use technique which can have notable results for PTSD, according to Paul Lynch, EFT founding master, advanced practitioner and research team volunteer with EFT International, the professional body for the practice of EFT:

> EFT is a technique that combines modern psychology with the traditions of acupuncture... I have worked with PTSD since 2008 and again and again I have seen EFT resolve PTSD where other treatments have failed. With EFT we have a highly effective, and gentle, treatment for trauma, literally at our fingertips.[20]

Research shows that stimulation of the end points of energy meridians, as in acupuncture, sends calming signals to the brain, lowering

---

20 Lynch, n.d.

cortisol.[21] In 2018, the UK medicines watchdog NICE officially recommended further investigation of EFT to treat PTSD in adults,
after NICE's own analysis showed it to be consistently within the
top four most effective and cost-effective interventions for PTSD.[22]
Paul Lynch says the power of EFT should not be underestimated:

> An EFT session can often bring relief from singular traumatic events
> in minutes. Complex cases take longer, but with commitment on
> behalf of the sufferer, relief from the debilitating effects of trauma
> are often accomplished even after one session... EFT allows you to
> hold the trauma at a distance. It can be represented by an image
> or a flashback, and you can tap on this image, and gradually clear
> the emotions it inspires, until the feelings of anger, fear, guilt and
> sadness abate.[23]

Havening

Havening comes from the word 'haven', meaning a safe space. This
is a simple technique we can all employ with our clients. I use it regularly with my grief coaching clients, my wellbeing coaching clients,
and even my nutritional therapy clients too when appropriate, suggesting they continue to use it on their own, outside of our sessions.
Havening is a touch therapy that can help to reduce anxiety. There
are plenty of YouTube videos to be found showing the techniques.
The way I was shown how to use it was to place each hand on the
opposite shoulder and make downward strokes from the shoulders
to the elbows, repeating certain phrases such as 'I am here, I am
safe, this is now' whenever you find yourself feeling your anxiety is
increasing or that you're reliving a traumatic event. Ask your client
to choose the phrases that resonate best with them. As we know, in
cases of PTSD, the mind doesn't always know the difference between

---

21 Church and Feinstein, 2007
22 NICE, 2018a; NICE, 2018b, p.287
23 Lynch, n.d.

a thought and something that's actually happening, and so when we remember the trauma, we really can be reliving it; therefore using words in the present tense together with the physical strokes can help bring us into the now.

According to Havening Techniques:

> The Havening Techniques are a healing modality that is designed to help individuals overcome problems that are the consequence of traumatic encoding... The Havening Techniques can be used within a psychotherapeutic setting with professional mental health care clinicians who have been fully trained and certified in The Havening Techniques. In addition, The Havening Techniques can be used by non-licensed practitioners as a protocol for coaching sessions.[24]

This is a simple and effective tool we can all use when we see any client who has experienced a trauma.

Aromatherapy, reflexology and massage

If you are an aromatherapist, massage therapist or reflexologist, then you will already know how these therapies can calm the nervous system and potentially help your client release some of the physical symptoms they may have due to grief and/or trauma, as well as the inevitable emotional build-up. These treatments provide enjoyable experiences, and this is undoubtedly to be welcomed during grief and trauma. As previously mentioned, traumatized survivors of 9/11 cited that massage was one of the therapies that helped them the most.

All 'touch therapies' have the potential to trigger an emotional response, so being a practitioner who is trauma-informed and grief-aware is vital. Those of us who aren't aromatherapists or reflexologists can signpost our clients to these therapies as gentle respite from the sometimes endless, soul-wrenching misery of grief and PTSD.

---

24 Havening Techniques, n.d.

Somatic therapy

Somatic healing is another body-centred approach for treating PTSD. Rather than focusing only on thoughts or emotions associated with a traumatic event, it addresses natural bodily (somatic) responses. It was first conceptualized by trauma therapist Dr Peter Levine in the 1970s, and over the years it has come to be considered a leading-edge therapy for PTSD. It helps to develop a deeper understanding of the mind/body connection, to improve the ability to release and regulate emotions and to build resilience.

Dr Levine believed that humans possess the capacity to release physical energy from stress but often thwart it by 'keeping it together' following trauma.[25] He believed that the ability to override the feelings felt during the traumatic event is what can lead to PTSD. Rather than just talk about the traumatic event, somatic therapists guide patients to focus on their underlying physical sensations. From there, the mind/body exercises may include breathwork, meditation, visualization, massage, grounding, dance and/or sensation awareness work. A slight word of caution regarding all claims made about treatments for PTSD: the trauma that stems from the death of a loved one may be considerably more complex and far reaching than some other traumatic events and therefore the level of success may vary and it could, at the very least, take more time before improvement is seen.

This chapter is perhaps best summed up by Bessel Van Der Kolk: 'Trauma treatment is not about telling stories about the past. Trauma treatment is about helping people to be here now, to tolerate what they feel right in the present.'[26]

---

25   Levine, n.d.
26   Van Der Kolk, 2014

CHAPTER 5

Mind, Body and Spirit

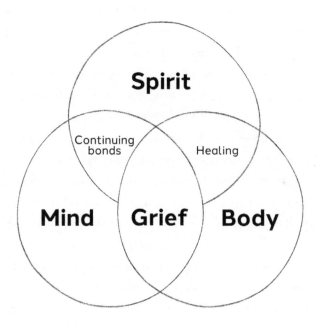

You should now have a good understanding about how grief varies greatly for each individual, depending on a multitude of factors. Grief can truly affect all aspects of ourselves – mind, body and spirit – and this is so often overlooked in mainstream approaches to grief. Developing this understanding can, I believe, make us more effective and open-minded practitioners, and enable us to bring something really quite noteworthy to the table, enabling us to better help our grieving clients. We've looked at the impact grief can have on a client's physical and mental health, but grief can sometimes change someone on a spiritual level, too, and, unlike the detrimental effects upon the mind and body, grief can, by contrast, sometimes actually have a positive and metamorphic effect upon the spirit.

Spirituality involves the belief that there is something greater than ourselves as just human beings with sensory experiences; that we are part of something much bigger and beyond our limited comprehension; that we are souls having a human experience, as Wayne Dwyer said,[1] with the implication that the soul continues after physical death. It may be that you hold some form of spiritual belief yourself, or it may be that you're an atheist or don't consider yourself to be a 'spiritual' person at all – and that's absolutely fine. But your grieving client may have found that an existing or newly found spiritual belief helps propel them forward into their new post-loss world that they might otherwise struggle with more acutely. If this is the case, then it's going to be really important that they feel their views are accepted and not in any way dismissed or minimized, regardless of their practitioner's own belief system.

In my grief coaching practice, I have been surprised by just how many clients want to talk about and are keen to explore their (often new-found) belief in an afterlife. Many like to share the dreams and signs they feel they have had from their loved one and are often keen to acquire knowledge of online resources or any books on the subject (see Chapter 10). Sadly, however, I am not particularly surprised when they tell me how they have picked up a sense of discouragement to pursue this (even if not necessarily explicit) from bereavement counsellors or therapists, as well as sometimes friends and family, with the implication that they are deluded in some way due to the intensity of their grief. This then makes them wary to communicate their views – and that's not ideal. So, if you share their belief, then please allow them to express how they feel, as this could provide a rare moment of upliftment for them in the midst of their grief and

---

1   Dwyer, 1989

could have a beneficial effect on the healing work you are doing with them. If you don't share their beliefs, then just listen without any hint of judgement that they could pick up on (be warned that grief can make some people extra sensitive). Life is hard enough for your grieving client without sensing any disapproval or negativity regarding what may be a surprisingly positive aspect of their grief.

It should also be noted, however, that you may also come across bereaved people who held some type of faith prior to a tragic loss but then go on to lose it as a result of what has happened to them, and others who have a religious faith that may preclude an ongoing spiritual connection with their loved one but may provide them with the sustenance they need to carry on. Whatever your grieving client's spiritual or religious beliefs, it goes without saying that they need to be acknowledged with respect.

It is estimated that a notably high percentage of bereaved people believe they have had one or more after-death communication (ADC) within a year of bereavement and, according to Raymond Moody MD, PhD, 75 per cent of bereaved parents believe they have had a communication from their child.[2] It seems possible perhaps that that the trauma and intensity of a significant loss can open you up and lead, in some cases, to a spiritual awakening that facilitates this communication. Here are a few quotes on spirituality and the afterlife from scientists:

Carl Sagan, astronomer and astrophysicist, said: 'Science is not only compatible with spirituality; it is a profound source of spirituality.'[3]

Albert Einstein said: 'Everyone who is seriously involved in the pursuit of science becomes convinced that some spirit is manifest in the laws of the universe, one that is vastly superior to that of man.'[4]

Gary E. Schwartz, PhD, director of the University of Arizona's Laboratory for Advances in Consciousness and Health, a former

2   Moody, 1993
3   Sagan, 2008
4   Calaprice, 2002

assistant professor at Harvard and tenured professor at Yale, says: 'Speaking as a scientist, I am now 99.9 percent certain that life continues after bodily death.'[5]

What may be of particular relevance to you if you're working with a bereaved client is that several studies have shown that those who believe in an afterlife and/or hold strong spiritual beliefs fare better in the grieving process than those who don't. Belief in an afterlife may help someone cope better with the death of a loved one, providing a sense of meaning during a time of despair and fostering continued emotional attachments with the person who has died. A study in the *BMJ* (*British Medical Journal*) concluded: 'People who profess stronger spiritual beliefs seem to resolve their grief more rapidly and completely after the death of a close person than do people with no spiritual beliefs.'[6] Although I don't think it's necessarily true that every type of grief is always resolved or indeed with any rapidity, I do feel, speaking from my own experience, that the development of a belief that this life isn't all there is and that energy or a soul continues in a different form can certainly help some of us survive a traumatic loss. This is perhaps a concept that is easier to comprehend for those who find that life is no longer as it was and that all you previously thought to be reality is thrown into question.

The kind of shift that occurs after a profound loss can undoubtedly sometimes lead to a searching for a way to connect to the person who has died, and, for some, mediums can facilitate this link, offering confirmation that a loved one's spirit is still around them, as well as reassurance that they are okay. As you can imagine, this has the potential to alleviate some of the suffering associated with grief. Of course, this will depend on finding a genuine and skilled medium. It's certainly a controversial area, and there is no doubt that grief does leave a person vulnerable and sometimes desperate for anything that might make them feel better in any way. This doesn't just apply

---

5   Pitstick, 2006, p.66
6   Walsh *et al.*, 2002

to seeking the services of a medium, however, but to looking for any type of therapist or practitioner who your grieving client might believe, due to any claims made, has the means to ease their suffering. For some, a positive experience with a medium is considerably more effective at easing the pain of bereavement than conventional psychological or counselling techniques. According to author and well-respected medium Claire Broad,[7] people often turn to mediums because the spiritual element is unacknowledged in traditional bereavement counselling, so there is clearly a need here that is not being met.

I concur with social worker Beth Christopherson who says:

Mediums who have a defined code of ethics and practice evidential mediumship, can be a valuable option of healing for those with grief. Mediumship is a resource that some clients already seek on their own, and it is one to which therapists could refer clients as a non-psychotherapeutic, spiritual resource. Clients receiving evidential mediumship can result in less fear of death, more peace or closure with unresolved issues with the departed, and a sense of comfort in the belief that the departed continue to support the living.[8]

A 2017 study entitled 'Exploring the effects of mediumship on hope, resilience, and post-traumatic growth in the bereaved' concluded:

Findings suggested that mediumship appeared to furnish some resilience. Coping which appears linked to hope, linked to post-traumatic growth and also appears to be enhanced when someone experiencing a sitting with a medium believes they have had confirmation of survival of the deceased. Hope appeared to be increased, and resilience and coping were reported as strengthened after a subjectively

---

7   Claire Broad, personal communication
8   Christopherson, n.d.

meaningful sitting with a medium. The implication therefore is that mediumship appeared to offer positive psychological tools to enable better coping styles post-bereavement.[9]

The Windbridge Institute[10] is currently conducting clinical studies on mediumship and its effects on grief. This and other studies will inform both the benefits and any potential risks from having a medium reading. As Beth Christopherson says:

> When mental health providers are not assessing the belief or hope in an afterlife, and providing additional options that incorporate this belief, an opportunity for more comprehensive healing benefits is lost. The widespread belief in the afterlife, as reflected in national survey data and in the popularity of shows on mediumship and ghosts, demonstrates the core need of many to explore the afterlife as part of their belief and coping system. Moving forward, a collaborative effort between grief scholars, afterlife researchers, and clinicians would beneficially inform best practices for integrating afterlife resources into grief treatment. The elephant in the room of grief should be directly addressed, as it leads to more healing options and addresses the core of the suffering of grief for so many. Grief is often described as a pit, but it does not necessarily have to be bottomless.[11]

As wellness practitioners, we could certainly participate in 'integrating afterlife resources into grief treatment'. And while your entire session may not be taken up by discussing spirituality and the afterlife with your client, it may prove useful to be aware of this far from insignificant aspect of their healing, if applicable to them.

Spirituality is undoubtedly one way of making sense of the world and of who you are after you have experienced a bereavement. If you

9   Cox, Cooper and Smith, 2017, p.6
10 www.windbridge.org
11 Christopherson, n.d.

have your own spiritual beliefs, then this may assist you in building rapport and trust with your client and opening up a discussion, obviously without imposing your own views, which may then help engender this potentially positive way of moving through grief. Your grieving client may be surrounded by friends and family who think that a belief that they will see their loved one again or that they receive signs from them is unhealthy in some way and needs to be discouraged. This leads the griever to feel a level of shame which is far from helpful, especially considering their circumstances. Non-judgemental acceptance of their views from us will mean a lot, particularly if they feel otherwise alone in their beliefs. And please remember that it may just be that the spiritual dimension of their loss is what is literally enabling them to go on living.

I spoke in Chapter 2 about avoiding the reframing of any 'negative' statements made by grieving clients who, after experiencing a devastating loss, might say, 'I'll never get over this' or 'This will never get better'. Actually, my own personal experience, and my experience of working with grieving clients, is that one way forward from these (understandable) feelings of hopelessness is the belief that our loved ones still remain close to us. If we are open to this idea, then we may start to feel them and receive communication from them, whether in the form of signs, through dreams or by finding thoughts randomly popping into our minds. Grief can feel dense physically, emotionally and energetically so the griever may need to raise their energetic vibration (through practices such as meditation or visualization) in order to receive this type of communication. This isn't always easy but if they're able to shift and lighten their energy, they may develop a belief that there are unseen connections that bond one soul to another, regardless of where they may be, and this can help to instil a sense of peace and hope. If your client has that, then it's possible they may find a way to live a meaningful life again, facilitated by moving *with* the person they have lost. They are able to let go of the fear that they are somehow leaving them behind. Above all, it just feels so much better to believe the people you have lost still walk beside you and that you are still able to love them and they are still able to love you – not in the past tense but in the here and now. It doesn't mean if you believe this that you leave all the pain of grief behind, but it may just mean you intersperse a terrible loss (or losses) with some brighter days of light and hope and an eye-opening view of the bigger picture.

CONTINUING BONDS

We will return to the continuing bonds theory later in the book, but we will touch on it here in relation to the mind, body and spirit. In *Answers from Heaven*, Theresa Cheung and Claire Broad say: 'The continuing bonds model demonstrates that the key to getting past grief is recognising that your relationship with the deceased isn't over, it has just changed. What was once physical is now spiritual.'[12] Of course, not all your bereaved clients will relate to this, but the ones that run with this idea can use it as a way to propel themselves through their grief.

Rather than being perceived as being in denial or as some kind of wishful thinking, the continuing bonds theory is thought to help a bereaved person to cope with their grief in a more constructive way. In fact, this theory is now considered by many as the healthiest way to grieve, and the idea that we should 'let go', 'move on' or 'find closure' is considered outdated and a psychologically damaging approach to grief. The continuing bonds theory is about finding ways to gradually adjust and redefine your relationship with the person you have lost, continuing your bond with them throughout your life and finding different ways to connect with them. Retaining the link with them rather than relinquishing it can enrich the life of the bereaved. To be clear, this doesn't necessarily have to mean spiritually, although for some obviously it does.

For generations, bereaved people were expected to stoically get

---

12   Cheung and Broad, 2017, p.307

over a loss, the implication being that after a certain time frame they should stop feeling sad, no longer voice their feelings and instead put on a brave face for the world. To all intents and purposes, most grievers did what was expected of them and gave a very good impression of having overcome their grief. This, in many cases, may have been far from the truth of the matter, and, as we know, the body keeps the score and if emotions are suppressed this can lead on to all kinds of issues.

In *Continuing Bonds: New Understandings of Grief*,[13] the authors question the linear models of grief, which are still used by many therapists, and which imply that the bereaved need to go through all the stages of grief before they can eventually reach acceptance. Unfortunately, this denies the reality of how people really grieve, which is rarely in a linear way. The continuing bonds theory suggested a new paradigm, rooted in the observation of healthy grief that does not resolve by detachment from the person who died, but instead by creating a new relationship that has been redefined and is ongoing. The continuing bonds theory normalizes the natural human attachment many feel, even in death. As Mitch Albom puts it: 'Death ends a life, not a relationship.'[14]

It may perhaps, on the face of it, look as though this theory could possibly encourage someone to remain stuck in their grief, living some kind of half-life, entombed with the memory of their dead person, preventing them from living their life to the full, but in fact the opposite is usually the case. *Continuing Bonds: New Understandings of Grief* and the research that has followed provide examples of how to continue the bond in a healthy way, without remaining stuck. In Chapter 10, I will outline a few ideas I have implemented both personally and with my clients which you may like to pass on to your own clients as a positive way of 'moving forward', as opposed of 'moving on'.

---

13 Klass, Silverman and Nickman, 1996
14 Albom, 2009, p.174

It's quite possible your grieving client will have heard of the five stages of grief, which we will be looking at more closely in Chapter 7, either from books, online sources or a bereavement counsellor or therapist they may have worked/be working with. Unfortunately, the old school thinking of encouraging detachment and letting go continues to prevail with some therapists and psychologists. However, the continuing bonds theory has changed the way most modern 'grief experts' view grief, so this will eventually filter through to everyone who works in the field. Certainly, those who actually experience grief are very likely to feel relieved that they are no longer expected to go through grief in linear way, get over their loss as soon as possible and be made to feel there's something wrong with them if doing all of this proves to be a struggle. To conclude, the continuing bonds theory allows a relationship to continue, which conversely can free the griever to engage in life again. This is to our advantage as wellness practitioners, as our client is subsequently more likely to then engage in our suggestions for healing.

SPIRITUAL BYPASSING AND TOXIC POSITIVITY

For all the potentially positive aspects of spirituality and the continuing bonds theory that we have looked at in this chapter, we now move on to the flipside of how these might hinder someone who is grieving. A spiritual bypass, or spiritual bypassing (a term coined by John Welwood, a Buddhist teacher and psychotherapist), is a 'tendency to use spiritual ideas and practices to sidestep or avoid facing unresolved emotional issues, psychological wounds, and unfinished developmental tasks'.[15] It may be useful to observe whether your grieving client is falling prey to this and, while this may not apply to you personally, some wellness practitioners do unfortunately have a tendency to encourage this practice themselves.

Many well-known spiritual or motivational 'gurus' advocate

---

15 Fossella, 2011

concepts such as 'choose happiness' and 'positive vibes only'. This relentless quest to be happy, particularly prevalent in certain areas of social media with its emphasis on only 'good' emotions and its disregard of the 'bad' ones, is clearly problematic for those experiencing grief. Dismissing very valid human emotions as 'negative' is known as 'toxic positivity'. I found this to be a real issue and ended up unfollowing a lot of the above-mentioned advocates of what often seems like positivity at all costs. Unsurprisingly, I couldn't find the silver lining in the death of my child. If something tragic has happened to you, the mindset that we are responsible for what we attract into our lives and that 'our thoughts become our reality' is supremely unhelpful, not to mention simplistic, naïve and downright insulting. Many who work in wellness buy into this, as I myself did to some extent before my son's death. I now see how astoundingly insensitive and very damaging this can be.

Unfortunately, there are wellness practitioners out there (and I have come across them personally) who will minimize someone's experience of grief. A responsible, proficient and wise practitioner (or, indeed, spiritual or motivational speaker) will never 'grief shame', imply that someone 'manifests' their experience of tragedy or loss, or suggest that anyone should either deny or 'rise above' their grief through some kind of spiritual practice or positive thinking at the expense of working through grief in a gentle, healthy and healing way.

CHAPTER 6

Case Studies

In this chapter, I give examples of how I have worked with some of my grieving clients. As you will see, they have all experienced different types of loss and secondary losses. They presented with a variety of physical and emotional symptoms, the commonality between them being that, to a large extent, these symptoms stem from their grief. I often begin by using my holistic grief wheel. You will see an example of this with Jodie's case study and you can read more about using the wheel in Chapter 10. Sometimes I see grieving clients without any nutritional therapy input, but below I demonstrate how I combine both holistic grief coaching with nutritional therapy. Your skill set may be different to mine, so these examples are just to illustrate how grief might present itself and so that you can take anything useful that might inform how you could approach your own sessions with a grieving client. All names have been changed.

OLIVIA, 19
Circumstances
Olivia's mother died when she was 18

Reasons for seeking help
Poor diet and lifestyle, hormonal issues, mood

Olivia's mother died of breast cancer when Olivia was doing her A levels. She lives with her dad and younger sister. Olivia had planned to go to university but decided to defer her place after the loss of her mum. However, with nothing planned in advance for her gap year, her life lacked structure and she lived a party lifestyle, involving binge drinking as a way to 'drown her sorrows'. Olivia's dad became concerned about her and subsequently sought both my help and also that of a psychotherapist.

Assessment at the first consultation

Olivia presented as confident and outgoing. She made no mention of her mother's death, so I followed her lead and we instead focused on her physical symptoms. I was aware that she had a therapist and was therefore able to assume that she was talking to them about her grief. Olivia said she experienced terrible PMT with sore breasts, skin outbreaks, moodiness and irritability, as well as heavy periods. She told me that 2–3 weeks of every month were dominated by her hormones. Olivia worked part-time as a waitress and, after getting up late and skipping breakfast, she would often eat mid-afternoon and then, after her waitressing shift, she would pick up some fast food at around midnight. On the days she didn't work, she would socialize in the evenings, drinking with friends, and would again often pick up something to eat on the way home. Her late lunch tended to be a cheese or ham sandwich with crisps or some pasta with pesto, followed by some chocolate or biscuits. Further enquiry revealed she suffered from constipation and that she could sometimes feel quite low.

I explained to Olivia that her hormonal symptoms most probably stemmed from her diet and lifestyle, as she was unlikely to be getting the nutrients she needed. I explained that even though she did eat, the quality of her food meant that she was most likely malnourished to some extent. This shocked Olivia. I reassured her that we could improve this significantly with changes to her diet and lifestyle, together with some supplements, if she was prepared to make these changes. I had already discovered there had always been some tendency towards hormonal imbalance since starting her periods aged 13, though nowhere near as bad as she currently experienced, but I then asked her when it was that this change in diet and lifestyle had occurred. She told me it was after her mother had died, which obviously hadn't been hard to work out. I didn't push this as I sensed she was guarded on the subject, but I did gently ask what kind of diet she had had when her mum was alive. As expected, it was significantly better, with regular meals and a relatively healthy packed lunch for school. At the end of the first session, I could see that I would need to tread carefully and remain focused on the physical symptoms, avoiding the elephant in the room – the pain of her loss – at least for now.

Suggested course of action

As it was Olivia's father who had set up the sessions, I needed to establish just how onboard Olivia was with making changes. I reassured her that I had helped a lot of other young women with hormonal issues and that I felt it would be fairly straightforward to improve this, but only if she was prepared to follow what I would be suggesting. Olivia wasn't prepared to give up drinking, which I had anticipated, but we agreed that, going forward, she would always eat before she went out in the evening and that she would try to reduce her alcohol intake by drinking spritzers, as well as trying to have at least two alcohol-free days a week.

As Olivia's current lifestyle meant she got up late and skipped breakfast, we agreed she would set an alarm and get up a bit earlier than she had been doing. As she said she couldn't face 'solid food', she agreed that she would try a smoothie of blueberries, half a banana, a tablespoon of almond butter, some plain yogurt and oat milk. I was encouraged when she came up with the idea of making it the previous evening before she went out so it was there ready in the morning, as this showed a certain amount of self-awareness that she might not make it otherwise. As well as discussing lunch ideas, we also discussed simple meals she could eat before she went out, such as an omelette with tomatoes, mushrooms and spinach, or some chicken or salmon that could be added to her regular staple of pesto and pasta (now to be whole-wheat) with a salad on the side. She agreed that she would try to eat five portions of vegetables a day and cut out the biscuits, although she was very pleased when I said she could have a little dark chocolate after her lunch. Finally, I recommended a women's multi vitamin and mineral supplement, which provided a good level of zinc and methylated B vitamins, as well as a probiotic to support gut health that may have been impacted by alcohol, poor diet and the stress from her bereavement.

Follow-up sessions

I wasn't sure how compliant Olivia would be, but, in fact, she surprised me. I had gathered that her dad worked long hours and got the impression that he was quite 'hands off'. He would also be dealing with his own grief. However, Olivia said he had been very encouraging about her dietary and lifestyle changes, and had even reinstated the family Sunday lunch for the first time since his wife had died. It's very common in grieving families that, once past the initial weeks when there is a certain unity, everyone then tends to grieve individually, which can lead to sense of separation and disconnect. It sounded as though this may have been the case in Olivia's family. It was therefore a positive sign, on many levels, that they were coming together for Sunday lunch.

At the second session, Olivia reported feeling more energetic (not something she had previously talked about as being a particular problem), having clearer skin and that her bowels were moving much better. Although she had had a period since her first session with me four weeks prior to this one, there had been no noticeable change in her PMT symptoms or the heaviness of her menstrual flow. I explained it may take a few cycles before she would see a significant difference. Olivia really loved her morning smoothie and we talked about how she could vary it. She was also eating before she went out or before a shift and now rarely picked up fast food on her way home. The reduction in her drinking was less successful, so I explained how alcohol adversely affects hormones and blood sugar balance and how it can deplete certain nutrients. She seemed to take this in. She admitted that she didn't always enjoy drinking and sometimes suffered with hangovers, so I asked if she was aware of what had led to her drinking beyond what felt enjoyable, and she went quiet. Again, I didn't want to push, so, even though I felt I was gaining her trust, I swiftly moved on. I knew Olivia made the link between her mother's death and drinking too much, so I would have to have faith that eventually she might be ready to address this.

At the third session, Olivia told me that her period had been slightly lighter and that she felt her PMS wasn't quite as bad as usual. Her dad and sister said she was less irritable and moody. I told her this was great news and that if she kept up the dietary changes and took the supplements, there was no reason that this couldn't improve further. She had even had four days in a row without alcohol and said she felt a lot better for it. She told me that she really wanted to 'get her s**t together' before she finally started university. I wanted to tell her how proud I thought her mum would be of her – but I resisted!

At the start of our fourth session, Olivia was clearly upset and didn't try to hide it with the mask she had clearly adopted in order to protect herself and to be able to function in the world. I asked her if she wanted to tell me what the matter was but that it was fine if she didn't. She said it was the anniversary of her mum's death the next day and that she'd also had a row with her dad that morning. She began to cry as she told me how much her family had changed and how they each just lived their own lives since her mum had passed away. I acknowledged how upsetting this must feel and then explained that her family wasn't alone in this and how everyone grieves differently, that there is no right or wrong way to do grief. Sometimes it's just important to normalize the impact of grief.

She continued to cry, telling me how close she and her mum were and how much she missed her. I asked her if she had heard of the continuing bonds theory; she hadn't, so I explained it to her. Following on from this, I then asked her if there was anything she might like to do the next day to honour her mum. She said she planned to visit her grave with some flowers and that the argument with her dad had been because Olivia wanted them to all go together as a family. We talked about how she would go home and explain calmly to her dad just how important it was for her and her sister that they all go to the church together. I asked her what kind of flowers she was going to buy, and she said she hoped to find some white roses, which had been her mum's favourite. We also talked about lighting a candle for her mum and buying a rose quartz crystal in her memory, as other ways to mark the day. As we drew the session to a close, Olivia told me that every night before she goes to sleep, she tells her mum she loves her.

The next time I saw Olivia, she informed me that she had let her dad know how important it was for them to visit her mum's grave together. Her sister had joined the conversation, and although there had been tears, Olivia said it got some things out in the open and that they did, in fact, all go together in the end. We talked about how good it was that she had been able to express her feelings to her dad and that her viewpoint was respected. She also acknowledged how hard it had been to watch him fall apart after her mother's death and how insecure this had made her feel, having always perceived him to be strong and invincible. Although it was good that Olivia was talking more freely about the loss of her mother, we eventually moved on to discuss her nutritional therapy progress, having not really discussed it during the previous session. Her hormones were definitely becoming more balanced and she felt she was not quite as low (which we agreed could have been down to clearing the air with her dad and getting past the anniversary, which she had naturally been dreading). Although her diet wasn't perfect, it was definitely a lot better than when I first saw her, and although the drinking was still more than ideal, I focused on all the positive progress she'd made.

Olivia had one more session with me, and progress continued to be made with her hormones, mood, skin and the continued absence of constipation. The majority of her month was definitely no longer completely dominated by her hormones, as she had reported at her first consultation. I told her she would now need to keep up her good work when she went off to university, and we left it that she would check in with an email in a few months' time. I was really impressed by Olivia's commitment at a time when life was particularly difficult for her. I'm quite certain her mum would be extremely proud of her.

SARAH, 53
Circumstances
Bereaved mother

Reasons for seeking help
Grief, insomnia, fatigue, anxiety

During the course of a discovery call, set up to establish what Sarah most needed help with, she told me that she was a newly bereaved mother experiencing insomnia, fatigue and anxiety. This was just five weeks after her 17-year-old daughter died suddenly from an undiagnosed heart condition. Sarah was understandably feeling completely overwhelmed with grief, as well as shouldering the additional responsibility for how her 15-year-old son was coping with the loss of his sister. Sarah is a single mother. She had seen her GP who offered antidepressants, which she was reluctant to take. She had been put on a waiting list for bereavement counselling. Sarah was devastated by her loss and felt alone and unsupported.

Assessment at the first consultation

Understandably, Sarah appeared to still be numb with shock and seemed to have many symptoms that suggested PTSD, although this had not been formally diagnosed. Immediately after her daughter's death, she didn't sleep at all for three days. She was unable to eat, felt nauseous and couldn't stop shaking. When I first met her, she was still experiencing many of these symptoms, together with flashbacks. She was also still very much on 'high alert'. I was able to reassure her that that this is a normal response to extreme shock. I explained that during trauma the nervous system goes into overdrive and that stress hormones are released as part of the fight-or-flight response because the body thinks it's in danger. I explained that shock is fundamentally a protective mechanism, and that it stops you from having to deal with the full impact of the emotional trauma. Sarah was coming to me for holistic grief coaching, so we would be looking at all aspects of her grief. Addressing bodily symptoms can give clients experiencing grief and trauma a much-needed glimmer of hope that it might be possible to feel better than they currently do, at least physically. Of course, the bigger issue is inevitably the heavy weight of their emotional pain, but working on the physical issues provides a tangible focus that can be very helpful.

After reassuring Sarah that I had some ideas for calming the physical manifestations of her traumatic loss, we spent the remainder of the first session talking about her daughter. My first question is always: 'What were they like?' Sarah's face lit up when I asked her this, and she went on to tell me about her daughter, which then naturally led on to her telling me about the pain of now living on without her. By the end of this session, I felt we had established a rapport which would be especially crucial to the sensitive nature of the work we would go on to do.

Suggested course of action

Sarah had lost half a stone within a week of losing her child as she couldn't stomach much food. She was now eating again but was still skipping some meals and mainly relying on takeaways and meals left for her by her neighbour, relieving her for now of the responsibility of shopping or cooking. Sarah barely left the house at this stage, so we discussed shopping online which meant she didn't need to face braving the supermarket and possibly bumping into people she knew, until she felt more ready. I discussed meals with her that wouldn't take too much of her currently precious energy. I explained the importance of blood sugar balance in her current state and suggested making meals as nutrient-dense as she could possibly manage. I explained that stress uses up nutrients and that grief is, inevitably, highly stressful. I suggested a specific supplement to calm the nervous system and help with sleep, together with a probiotic, as serotonin can be depleted during the grieving process and, as we know, serotonin is manufactured in the gut. I also added in a supplement that I have used with many clients over the years who experience low mood or depression, and Sarah was keen to try this instead of the antidepressants her GP had prescribed. In addition, I suggested trying breathing techniques, particularly before sleep when she got the flashbacks. We did these together during the consultation which, from experience, I have learned helps the likelihood of them being implemented at home. For the same reason, I taught her how to do havening to reduce the constant feeling of anxiety she said she was feeling. I suggested she did the technique as often as needed. I followed everything up succinctly in an email, keeping it simple, but knowing that, understandably, Sarah might not be able to hold on to all we had discussed. I was aware I had made quite a few suggestions, all of which I felt had the potential to help her in her extremely challenging circumstances. However, my hope at this stage was that she would just take what she most needed now and come back to the rest later.

Follow-up sessions

To her immense credit, Sarah made some of the suggested changes to her diet, having started to make simple balanced meals for herself and her son. Her appetite was gradually improving, which helped. She was taking her supplements, as directed, and she reported sleeping a little better and feeling less fatigued. She agreed that being proactive about your physical health gives you back a little control over your life at a time when you feel you no longer have any. However, these positive steps that Sarah had done so well to accomplish could in no way compensate for the raw pain of her loss, and during the second session, Sarah cried non-stop. It felt important to give her the space to just talk and tell her story without directing her in any way, but, at the end of the session, I suggested she tried journaling before our next session, as a way to possibly express and release some of her pain. I also recommended the book *It's OK That You're Not OK* by Megan Devine.[1] I made it clear that these suggestions were optional and to be taken only if they resonated with her as potentially helpful.

In the third session, we had a nutritional therapy check-in, and Sarah reported some further modest improvements, despite a few understandable fluctuations in compliance when the grief engulfed her. Her insomnia and fatigue were better than they were, but still there, and although she reported feeling less anxious in some ways, she still sometimes felt on 'high alert'. I adjusted her supplements to include one with a higher level of B vitamins and magnesium, plus omega 3 to help the brain fog, anxiety and depression, as well as benefiting the heart (see below), because she didn't eat much oily fish. I explained that she was doing incredibly well in taking my nutritional therapy suggestions on board but that some symptoms would take time to resolve, which was only to be expected after all she had been/was going through.

---

1   Devine, 2017

Sarah mentioned that she sometimes felt as if she couldn't breathe and that she would catch her breath. She couldn't understand why this was, but it had only happened since her daughter's death. I explained that although she must see her GP if this remained a cause for concern, this might possibly be because, in Traditional Chinese Medicine, the lungs are believed to be associated with grief and sadness. Symptoms of lung imbalance are thought to include shortness of breath and shallow breathing, depression and excessive crying. She said this made sense, and we agreed that grief manifests in ways you never think of until you go through it yourself. I asked her some questions about her heart and, without trying to worry her, explained that when you're emotionally broken-hearted, your heart can physically be affected, too. I was also aware that her daughter had died of an undiagnosed cardiac condition, although both Sarah and her son had now had genetic testing for this and appeared to be fine. She said that she wasn't experiencing any obvious symptoms but agreed to visit her GP if she noticed any. We discussed the fact that she was very traumatized and still in shock, and how child loss sometimes feels as if it will be impossible to survive because the pain is just so monumental.

Sarah hadn't tried journaling yet, although someone had bought her a nice notebook so she planned to, and she didn't feel up to reading yet as she was unable to concentrate. I recommended online grief yoga for the anxiety, and we then spent the remainder of the third session discussing her concerns for her son, how he wouldn't talk to her or anyone else about his sister's death, and how he couldn't cope when he saw Sarah visibly upset and would have to leave the house. As a single parent, this was an additional challenge that Sarah had to deal with.

Sarah reported back in the fourth session that she loved the grief yoga and said it really helped calm the anxiety. She was also finding journaling helpful as a way of processing her pain, too. In this session, we talked about the unforeseen practical issues that present themselves after a death, such as someone's social media presence and accessing their phone – dilemmas no mother ever considers they will have to address. Sarah also had huge anxiety over her daughter's possessions, feeling it would be impossible to get rid of anything that she had ever held or worn. I understood that this would feel like somehow shrinking the evidence of her child's existence. I reassured her that there was no pressure to sort through anything until she felt ready. Sarah said she felt she might never be ready, and I reassured her that if that was the case, then that was completely fine. However, I also told her that David Kessler says when we have to eventually shrink the outer evidence that our loved ones lived, we must increase the evidence within us. That we are the living, breathing evidence that they lived.[2]

I talked to her about the continuing bonds theory and how remaining connected to loved ones can help facilitate the ability of the bereaved to better cope with loss and the subsequent changes to their lives. Following on from this, I asked Sarah to consider ways she might like to honour her daughter, and we discussed various ideas, such as a memorial bench, planting a rose bush, raising money for charity in her daughter's name, etc. I suggested involving her son, asking him what he would like to do to honour his sister, as this might aid his healing process, too.

In later sessions, we began to talk a little about spirituality. Sarah had by now visited a medium and was amazed by some of the validations that the medium gave her and which she couldn't possibly have known. This comforted Sarah and, together with other information she was given, allowed her to believe that her daughter was okay and at peace. I went on to talk to Sarah about post-traumatic growth. Post-traumatic growth can, if we are able to allow it to, show us that pain can shift our perception of life and that there are several ways you can grow after a tragedy. These include discovering a new purpose in life, helping others who have

---

2   Kessler, n.d.

experienced a similar tragedy, becoming more compassionate, a deepening spirituality, discovering an inner strength you perhaps didn't know you had, and developing stronger relationships. While acknowledging that there are some losses you will never recover from, you can try to move forward into the future in the best way that you can, while carrying your loved one with you in your heart. Sarah liked this concept and impressed me with her ability to maintain hope for growth, healing and purpose as she lives on without her eldest child.

With a holistic grief coaching client who wants to include nutritional therapy, I usually suggest a programme of six sessions, which include an initial 90-minute consultation, followed by 60-minute sessions fortnightly, which will mainly be coaching with around 15–20 minutes of nutritional therapy, depending on what might be required. After the initial package of six, Sarah went on to have further sessions (to date, for over two years) where we check on her diet and adjust the supplements, and then go on to talk about her grief beyond the intense shock of the early months. The fact that I was also a bereaved mother definitely gave our sessions an added dimension that wouldn't have been there otherwise, and Sarah made me aware that this made an appreciative difference to her. We were in agreement that only another bereaved mother is going to truly understand what losing a child actually feels like.

Sarah remained concerned about her son, but he received some counselling via his school, which she thought had helped to some extent. Sarah decided not to pursue any additional support from bereavement counselling when she finally came to the top of the waiting list as she felt our sessions provided what she needed. However, she did, at my suggestion, find a local group for bereaved parents (The Compassionate Friends) which she found supportive. Although Sarah will never get over the tragic loss of her child, she is doing as well as she can under the circumstances. She is undoubtedly still processing her trauma and experiencing long-term depression. As with most bereaved parents, the grief remains intense and casts an inevitably long shadow. Life can never be the same again. However, focusing on her son's welfare has kept her going, as does her ongoing bond and spiritual connection with her daughter. Regular exercise and continuing with the healthy lifestyle she established during our early sessions also helps, along with our now less frequent sessions. Last but not least, Sarah has found a sense of purpose by fundraising for a charity for cardiac risk in young people, hoping this will one day mean fewer young people will die from an undiagnosed heart condition.

ANDREW, 76
Circumstances
Widower

Reasons for seeking help
Grief, chronic fatigue syndrome (CFS)

Andrew's wife died of Alzheimer's two years prior to his first consultation with me. He was retired and had two adult sons, whom he rarely saw. He was a quietly spoken, reserved man and presented as someone who withheld his emotions. His symptoms of CFS first appeared when his wife died. She had gone through a long illness which had clearly been extremely stressful and traumatic for him. Andrew initially came to me for grief coaching. On discovering his issues with CFS, we decided to address them with nutritional therapy, as well as continuing with some grief coaching sessions. Andrew had many of the symptoms linked to CFS, including insomnia, anxiety, IBS and brain fog, as well as debilitating fatigue. Many of these symptoms cross over with the symptoms we find in grief.

Assessment at the first consultation

It was clear straight away that, at this point, Andrew just needed someone to listen to his story. So that's what I did. It was quickly evident that he hadn't had anyone to talk to about his wife, her illness or her death, as he had a distant relationship (literally and emotionally) with his sons, one of whom lived abroad and the other hundreds of miles away in the Lake District. There didn't appear to be any other family, and he didn't seem to have many friends. It became evident that he lived a fairly isolated, insular life where he was free to ruminate on the loss of his wife and stress over his physical symptoms. It seemed that he and his wife were fairly enmeshed and, once he'd retired, did everything together. He described how although his wife had a diagnosis of Alzheimer's, he had struggled to face up to the fact that she would actually die, despite her deterioration. He went into great detail about every aspect of her illness and death. It seemed that he very much needed to share this with someone, although he talked about it in a very matter-of-fact, detached way. He told me that during his wife's final days he barely slept and lived on 'coffee and adrenaline'. I asked if he had felt 'tired but wired', and he said very much so.

When Andrew then told me how, once the funeral was over, he was overcome with exhaustion and couldn't get out of bed, I thought this would probably have been a fairly natural reaction to witnessing his wife's suffering and then experiencing the pain of her subsequent death. And I'm sure it was, in part. However, he was then beset by other issues, including a nasty cold virus he couldn't shake off and symptoms he had no major prior experience of, such as IBS, brain fog, headaches and insomnia. He admitted he became rather obsessional with these symptoms, especially as he couldn't understand why nothing improved with time. It seemed also that what he was experiencing physically was providing a distraction from the emotional weight of his grief.

I thought it sounded as though Andrew was dissociating, as

there was a sense of him being detached from what had happened to him and a disconnect between his body and his emotions. Although he told me about what had happened to him in great detail during the first session, he came across as emotionally detached from what he was telling me. When there's dissociation, the brain can't map the body clearly and so it sounds the alarm (see Chapter 4). My aim was, as much as I could, to help restore some of the integration between his body and brain so that the nervous system could regulate itself as it's meant to, which would then improve the symptoms he was experiencing.

I knew that there is often a tipping point with CFS, and his wife's lengthy illness and death could be seen as that final straw. There can also often be a virus that is difficult to shake off, which is something Andrew experienced. He had visited his GP, who mentioned ME/CFS to Andrew but told him to see if his symptoms improved; if they hadn't within three months, he could come back to see him. However, by that time, the pandemic had begun and, at the time of his session with me, Andrew hadn't seen his GP again because he felt there was little point as only urgent referrals were being made. I asked Andrew whether he would like to address these symptoms with a full nutritional therapy session next time, and he agreed that he would.

Suggested course of action

Although I was now aware of Andrew's very debilitating physical symptoms and possibly CFS, this first session was mainly focused on hearing about the loss of his wife and how it had impacted him. I explained how 'the body keeps the score' and that maybe his body was perhaps 'expressing' his grief because, as he had admitted, he had been in denial that she was actually going to die even while witnessing her very distressing decline. I felt it was positive that he had actually acknowledged he needed to talk about his loss and that he sought grief support. If I could help him recognize the link between his grief and how it may be a factor in the development of CFS, this might play a significant part in his healing – on all levels. Although Andrew appeared devoid of emotion as he talked, I felt that the first session was beneficial in simply allowing him to tell his story, in a way that I suspected he wouldn't have had the chance to do previously. In grief, we need to tell our story, sometimes many times over, in order to begin to process it.

Follow-up sessions

The next session was given over to nutritional therapy alone. While taking his case history, it became clear that Andrew had always been quite anxious about his health, stemming from a period in hospital as a boy for a mystery illness that was never diagnosed. He said that he didn't like school as he was badly bullied. He was an only child. His mother had suffered from anxiety and depression, and he had taken her death, from a stroke when he was 26, very hard. Soon after this, he met his wife who, it transpired, did everything for him. He worked hard and wasn't very involved in his sons' lives, although was clearly devoted to his wife. He admitted that he had probably suffered from anxiety all his life but hadn't really acknowledged it as 'it wasn't something that got talked about until recently'.

Aside from the 'mystery illness' in childhood, which I suspected was possibly psychosomatic as it was at the time of the bullying, there was little of any note in his health history, aside from glandular fever as a teenager, which is sometimes seen in people who go on to develop CFS. His diet was traditional meat and two veg when his wife was alive, and he had tried to keep this up after she died but admitted he sometimes felt too tired to get anything other than a sandwich or a bowl of cereal. He said he had lost weight since her death. As the IBS symptoms and the headaches had only been problematic since his wife's death, it seemed likely that an underlying cause of this could be the sympathetic nervous system dominance due to the trauma, as the sympathetic nervous system exerts a predominantly inhibitory effect upon the GI tract. With gut problems, there is often a dysregulation of the nervous system stemming from chronic stress. I felt that, alongside grief coaching to address the root cause, a nutritional therapy protocol that included avoiding wheat, dairy and sugar could also lead to an improvement in his digestive symptoms, as well as helping with the fatigue, too.

We discussed simple balanced meals he could make for himself and cutting down gradually on coffee so as not to suffer from withdrawal headaches. I decided on a supplement programme focusing first and foremost on calming the nervous system, as well as some aloe vera for his IBS symptoms, plus a probiotic, working on the premise that there was very likely to be sympathetic nervous system overactivity and parasympathetic dysfunction, and that this was probably the cause of the IBS, as well as his other symptoms. This dysfunction of the nervous system can be observed in cases of both traumatic grief and CFS. I also recommended an effective natural roll-on stick for his frequent headaches, which contains lavender and camomile, and explained how taking paracetamol so frequently would not be helpful for his liver and may even be causing subsequent headaches. He didn't appear too keen on trying the breathing techniques I suggested for his anxiety and insomnia, so I suggested a supplement that might help him sleep.

There is no doubt that there was a crossover to be seen in the symptoms of CFS and those of grief (this may be especially true in grief where we see notable stress caused by trauma). This crossover could be seen as complicating the way I approached Andrew. However, in many ways, it didn't really matter, at this stage, whether I was addressing the CFS or the grief, as I would fundamentally take the same approach. The difference would lie in how I worked with Andrew aside from the nutritional therapy.

As I had done some additional training in CFS/ME/fibromyalgia, I already had an understanding that recovery is possible if all aspects of health and wellbeing are looked at and the entire focus isn't just on addressing the physical symptoms. CFS, like grief, is complex. Many people who have CFS are thought to have certain personality traits, such as being highly sensitive, prone to anxiety, having perfectionist tendencies and being quite driven. The other aspects important to address for recovery from CFS include emotional health, environment, relationships and even having a life purpose. These aspects of health and wellbeing can also be applied to grief, as long as we view them, perhaps, as essential to 'healing' rather than essential to 'recovery' as we would with CFS.

The major difference is that although it is helpful to aspire to recovery with CFS, it's not especially helpful (as previously discussed) to use the word 'recovery' with grief, especially where the emotional impact of the loss has been great. You can recover from an illness, but grief is not an illness, so recovery is an inappropriate choice of word. However, as we have explored, it is possible for the suffering experienced in grief to lessen, and certainly it's very possible that many of the physical symptoms initially felt in early grief will decrease or eventually disappear. The more serious and far-reaching physical manifestations of grief we looked at in Chapter 3, such as PTSD, cancer, heart disease and a shortening of life expectancy, do not typically cross over with CFS, or at least not for the same reasons.

At his next consultation, Andrew had begun to make a little progress. He reported that his anxiety was a bit better and that his IBS was definitely showing signs of improvement. He felt that removing gluten from his diet had helped. He was still getting some headaches, but was trying to use the roll-on stick rather than paracetamol as much as he could. Because of his headaches and past history of glandular fever, I decided to add a supplement to provide liver support, as I thought this might be beneficial. The liver is considered to be the seat of the emotions, and so I felt this might also help with grief, and especially as he seemed to have some difficulty in expressing his emotions. There was something very 'held' about Andrew, and I felt supporting the organ of detoxi-fication might be helpful on an emotional as well as physical level.

The supplement I had suggested for sleep didn't seem to be making any difference, so I recommended an alternative, explaining that sometimes different things work for different people. There wasn't much change in his fatigue, but I explained it was early days and that it may take a little time. He was really making an effort with his diet, so I encouraged him to believe that this would eventually start to pay off with regard to energy levels, as it was starting to for the IBS and anxiety. In this consultation, we just talked about the physical, but I suggested we bring back in the grief work next time and he agreed. Before we finished, I said I was going to set him a task before the next session. I suggested that he wrote a letter to his wife, telling her everything he needed to say to her. Andrew didn't hold any spiritual or religious beliefs, but I explained that it was for him to get anything he needed to off his chest, rather than a 'communication' with her if this wasn't what he believed. I felt this exercise would give a little more structure to the grief coaching part of the forthcoming session, although I planned to let him just talk in a free-flowing way if it appeared this was what he needed.

At our next session, Andrew seemed to be a little more upbeat and expressed that he was beginning to feel hopeful that his health could improve. Progress was still modest, but he reported some improvement in all areas – fatigue, headaches, brain fog, insomnia and IBS. I told him it would take time and that a holistic approach to both CFS and grief were key, and I could see that he was beginning to understand this. We then moved on to the grief part of the session. He had written the letter to his wife, although he admitted that he had been reluctant to try this. However, he said he found it a surprisingly helpful exercise once he got going and wrote down what he had wanted to say to her but hadn't while she was alive. It was clear that he felt a certain amount of guilt and sadness for not being 'a good enough husband' and that he felt he hadn't been as demonstrative or as affectionate as he might have been. We talked about this, and it seemed that by doing so and through writing the letter, he might be starting to address some of the feelings that he was finding so difficult.

In later sessions, we changed some of the supplements and added in some CoQ10 to further support energy. Andrew continued to make progress with his physical symptoms. He was very pleased about this, but it became evident that his focus on the physical symptoms had distracted him to some extent from the devastating emotional impact of his loss, confirming my initial thoughts. It was quite challenging to get him to acknowledge this, and now that he felt he had 'told his story', he definitely preferred to focus on the physical where he could see measurable progress and because this was now an area of health that had become less uncomfortable for him. I decided to send him some information about EMDR as I thought this might be a suitable way for him to address the trauma associated with his wife's death, although he decided it wasn't something he wanted to pursue.

I persevered with trying to get him to open up more and connect with his emotions – sometimes he did and would then say how helpful it was to talk. I was aware that his old wounds from childhood and early adulthood (bullying, the mystery illness, the death of his mother) may be impacting both the grief felt for his wife and also the chronic fatigue too, but he was reluctant to explore this connection. I did, however, find a support group for widowers and recommended the benefits of talking to others in the same position. I had to gently prompt him a few times on this, but he did eventually go to a meeting. He now attends regularly, and this has been really quite significant for Andrew, both in terms of the CFS having improved sufficiently for him to go, and in terms of sitting in a room with other bereaved men and the emotional charge that this might bring with it.

Following the death of a partner, there are a lot of decisions to be made from the moment they have died; some are small and some are big, but all are now the sole responsibility of the remaining spouse, which can feel scary when you're used to relying on your combined experience, ideas and insights. Facing major decisions without anyone to lean on can feel daunting and destabilizing, especially at first when a bereaved partner can very much feel as if they've been thrown into the deep end with no lifebuoy in sight. To connect with others who have lost a partner, and so have also experienced all of this, can be really helpful.

The practical challenges of being newly alone can feel endless. Partners invariably share tasks – one may do the cooking and shopping, the other takes out the bins and looks after all the technology. Suddenly, the remaining partner is responsible for every task, as well as for the finances, which may have previously been shared. This can add another very significant layer of stress to an already very stressful time.

We generally don't even notice how much of a couple's world it is until we're no longer part of it, especially when it comes to going out to dinner or on holiday, for instance. Widows and widowers report that friends in couples hesitate to invite them to anything, worried that, as a single person, they will now feel out of place, which might be awkward for all concerned. The plans you might have had for your future together can no longer be realized and that can instil a sense of very deep sadness. Most marriages or partnerships (whether good or bad) operate and function as two people joining their lives together, so after the loss of a partner, the one who is left feels somewhat incomplete. There is an intrinsic need in most of us to have someone with whom we can share our deepest thoughts and feelings, and it is usually our partner who fulfils that need. In addition, it will also be the everyday mundane things that will be greatly missed, such as little in-jokes, eating a meal together or watching TV.

Loss of identity is therefore an issue you might observe if working with a widow/widower or anyone who has lost their partner. Because a partner often fulfils multiple roles, such as best friend, lover, peer, co-parent, confidant, someone with whom to share chores and financial decisions, the loss can feel colossal. It can feel overwhelmingly lonely, especially after a long marriage, as was the case with Andrew.

It's always easier in any type of coaching to work with clients who are emotionally open and have a certain degree of self-awareness, and Andrew was at times challenging in this regard. CFS can be notoriously difficult to address successfully, so I felt glad that he made such relatively good progress. I think his reserved nature and the bullying he experienced in childhood had left him guarded, so in some ways I felt honoured he let me in as much as he did. I appreciated that it was difficult for Andrew to even seek grief support in the first place, and so I have to commend him for being brave enough to do so.

JODIE, 31
Circumstances
Boyfriend died by suicide eight years ago

Reasons for seeking help
Stress, panic attacks

Jodie and her boyfriend, Joe, had met at school and were childhood sweethearts who began their relationship when they were both 15. Whereas Jodie came from a relatively secure background, Joe didn't, although he gained some stability from being included in Jodie's family meals and activities. He struggled academically, which increasingly affected his self-worth, and he began to get into trouble both in school and outside of school. However, he and Jodie believed that they were soulmates, and when they left school, they moved in together. For a while, everything seemed fine, but Joe's mental health began to slowly deteriorate, and he started to self-medicate using drugs and alcohol. Jodie stood by him, but it became increasingly difficult for her. Joe eventually lost his job, and Jodie never knew what state she might find him in when she got home. She tried unsuccessfully to get him help, and one day she returned home to find he had taken his own life.

Assessment at the first consultation

Jodie booked a nutritional therapy consultation with me, telling me at the time of booking that she needed help with stress and panic attacks. She had tried various therapies to address this over the years, but nothing had worked, so she wondered if looking at her diet might be the key. I took her case history, and she told me how work was a particular cause of her stress, but it wasn't until I got to asking if she had children or had ever been pregnant that she told me she and her boyfriend had planned to have children but that he had died eight years ago. I said how sorry I was to hear this and asked if she knew I was also a grief coach. She said she had read on my website that I was but had thought grief support was usually only for people who had lost someone more recently. I said that was not necessarily the case and asked if her boyfriend's death was still impacting her. She began to cry. I asked her if she would like to tell me about him, and she said she would. The rest of the consultation was given over to her talking to me about their love for each other and what had happened to him.

It was a heartbreaking story and one I hadn't anticipated hearing at the start of the consultation. It was clear Joe's loss was utterly devasting to Jodie, as well as to his mum, his friends and Jodie's family, who had loved him like one of their own. Jodie and Joe were both just 23 when he died, and the loss of a young person has an astonishing ripple effect, touching many people with its tragedy. Unfortunately, though, because Joe had died by suicide, Jodie had to deal in some instances with people's judgement, and so her grief was not only traumatic but had elements of being disenfranchised too, due to the regrettable stigma around suicide. Fortunately, Jodie had a supportive family, but she had struggled

– and still struggled – to deal with the loss of the person that she considered to be her soulmate, as well as with the indescribable trauma of finding his body. She also now, in addition, had to deal with people telling her it was time to move on and that she should be looking for another boyfriend by now.

Suggested course of action

As we had abandoned the nutritional therapy aspect of the consultation halfway through, I emailed Jodie the rest of the questions I had planned to ask so that she could return her replies to me prior to the next session. I asked her how she would like to go forward, and she said she would like to continue with some grief support but also with looking at her diet, too. I suggested that the next session we could combine both, and then we would decide how to go forward after that. I also sent her my holistic grief wheel.

Follow-up sessions

The answers I received from Jodie regarding the nutritional therapy questions, as well as her completion of the wheel, were very enlightening. For the holistic grief wheel, she scored herself 9 for both 'life purpose' and 'spiritual life' but only 3 for 'mental health'. (With 10 being the highest possible score and 1 the lowest.) I was interested to find out about more about this notable difference. It was pretty clear that the panic attacks were related to the trauma of Joe's death and her extreme shock at discovering his body. Although the panic attacks could be seemingly unrelated, they always happened when she felt she had no control, whether this was related to a work situation or her fear of losing other people she loved. She knew the panic was irrational and out of proportion to the situation, but it scared her that she felt she had no control over her emotional and bodily responses – which went back to the way she felt when discovering Joe's body.

Her panic attacks included a racing heart, sweating, shaking, feeling lightheaded and shortness of breath. She said that the dread and anticipation of having a panic attack, such as when she had to stand up and talk in front of others at work or when her mum didn't answer her phone, could send her spiralling and took her straight back to what she experienced in terms of physical symptoms when she had found Joe's body. The body remembered. Jodie had tried CBT, antidepressants and smoking cannabis among other things, but nothing helped for long. It seemed to me that she clearly had PTSD, despite the fact that this had never been actually diagnosed, and she suspected this herself. Jodie still had flashbacks sometimes, but never nightmares.

I suggested that she removed all caffeine, which might exacerbate her anxiety and panic attacks. I suspected she didn't drink enough water and that dehydration might be acting as an additional trigger for her anxiety panic attacks. I also explained that low blood sugar can mirror symptoms of anxiety or worsen them, so it was therefore important not to go too long without food and to ensure her meals were balanced. It turned out that because of her job she sometimes missed lunch and forgot to drink water, living instead on endless cups of tea throughout the day. I emphasized that making these changes could be significant. As well as a multi vitamin with a good level of B vitamins for stress, I recommended an omega 3 supplement (Jodie didn't eat oily fish) and an additional supplement containing magnesium, L-theanine and ashwagandha to help the anxiety and panic attacks.

When we moved on to the grief wheel during the second half of the session, I commented on how great it was that she scored 'life purpose' and 'spiritual life' so highly and I was interested to know the reasons for this. Jodie said that her job as a primary school teacher was very rewarding and that it gave her a definite sense of purpose and meaning. She worked at a lovely school, got on with all the staff, and had developed a good reputation as a teacher that parents wanted their children to be taught by, so she felt valued and appreciated. I was so pleased to hear that Jodie had something so positive in her life.

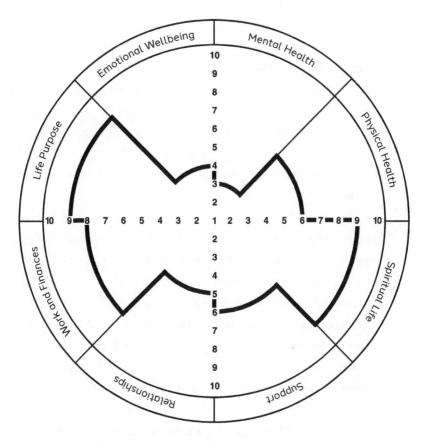

JODIE'S HOLISTIC GRIEF WHEEL (SEE CHAPTER 10 FOR
HOW TO USE THE HOLISTIC GRIEF WHEEL)

I then asked about the 9 she gave for spiritual life, and she told me this was because she knew Joe was still with her and that when she felt calm enough, she could feel him. I asked if this helped, and she replied that if she didn't have this strong feeling, she might not have been able to go on after he died. She told me about the signs she felt she had received from Joe and how he liked to mess with the lights in her flat, as well as her phone. I asked how others felt when she told them about this, and she replied that there was only one person she could talk to about her communications from Joe and who didn't dismiss what she believed to be true. She felt that some thought that this and her panic attacks just indicated that she was mentally unstable in some way. I reassured her that I believed her and that it was not uncommon. She agreed and told me she'd done lots of reading on the subject and was part of supportive online communities who share her beliefs, which helped her feel as though she wasn't going mad. She had also visited mediums several times over the past eight years and was firmly convinced that Joe was coming through loud and clear. She was also given validation that only she could have known about.

I really liked that Jodie was so direct and honest in every respect. I felt this attitude had helped her survive this tragedy in many ways, though obviously she was stuck in an anxiety loop which we would now attempt to break, in part through diet and supplements, as well as havening and yoga (I recommended Yoga with Adriene, which who has free online classes for PTSD and well as several for anxiety).[3] I also suggested breathwork, but Jodie had already tried this with one of the therapists she saw and said it hadn't helped. I felt havening might be an alternative approach, in addition to the online yoga which would involve breathwork in a different form. We also talked about specific essential oils that could help anxiety, providing a sense of wellbeing (see Chapter 10).

In subsequent sessions, it was clear Jodie had embraced everything I had suggested and was managing her stress a lot better. With the nutritional side underway, we used our sessions for coaching, allowing Jodie a safe space to talk about her darkest thoughts, her spirituality and her hopes for the future. In particular, we worked through Jodie's fear of meeting someone else and her guilt over the prospect of another man replacing Joe and of

---

3   https://yogawithadriene.com

leaving him behind in the past. She understood that these fears were playing into her anxiety and panic attacks, and keeping her stuck in this respect. Jodie journaled through a lot of these fears, which brought her clarity, especially when she wrote directly to Joe. It began to click that she didn't have to leave Joe behind and that forming another relationship didn't have to threaten what they'd had together. She could always keep Joe in her heart, and her belief in life after death meant that she would always have a relationship with him and that this didn't need to be in conflict with forming another partnership. They would be energetically different. She knew ultimately that Joe would want her to live a full life and to go on to have children, which was very much something she wanted.

Jodie was a pleasure to work with. She was open and willing to do the work, both in terms of nutritional therapy and, more importantly, when it came to her grief and the effects of trauma on her mental health and emotional wellbeing. I suggested an organization for bereaved people affected by suicide and also a few accounts to follow on Instagram, as I felt it might help her to find others in a similar position to hers and the very particular devastation of suicide. I felt great hope for Jodie and her future, and by the end of our sessions together, I know that she did, too.

JENNY, 43

Circumstances

Widow with two young children

Reasons for seeking help

Weight gain, depression

Although an enquiry email from Jenny mentioned only her weight gain and depression, a discovery call with her then revealed that a year ago her husband had died suddenly of a heart attack while playing football. He was 42. They had two young children, now aged six and four. Although she had always struggled with her weight, Jenny was now comfort eating and was classed as obese. The struggle of coping with the practicalities of life with two young children, alongside the shock and grief of her loss, had left her very depressed and experiencing suicidal ideation.

Assessment at the first consultation

It appeared that Jenny was experiencing a certain amount of delayed grief due to having sole responsibility for two young children and the demands that this brings at the best of times. In many ways, this was a distraction from the shock and grief she was enduring, but when her kids were at school, Jenny would crawl under the duvet and only force herself to get up at school pick-up time. I asked if she ever felt suicidal, and she said she did and would love to go to sleep and just not wake up, but she also said she had no choice but to go on as she couldn't let her children grow up without a mother and a father. I asked if she felt she was a danger to herself or others, and she said no, but I emphasized that she must seek help from her GP if that changed. I also gave her the phone number for the Samaritans. Although I would keep this to the forefront of my mind during our sessions, I felt that her suicidal ideation was a normal reaction to a terrible situation, and I made sure she felt no shame around feeling this way. I was as certain as I could be that Jenny's maternal instincts would override her desire to put a permanent end to her pain.

The first consultation revealed the extent of her comfort eating, which was mainly based around whole packets of biscuits or cakes when she retreated to her bed, along with a hot chocolate. Evenings, when the children were in bed and the full force of missing her husband was felt, were another trigger point. She also admitted to drinking around half a bottle of wine each evening, although I suspected this might be an underestimation. There were also takeaways, mainly pizza or Chinese, three or four times a week.

Jenny had planned to get a job once her youngest had started school (which he had now done) but she didn't feel ready. Her husband had life insurance and so financially Jenny was fine for the moment. Due to her poor diet and, no doubt, also her grief, Jenny experienced fatigue and digestive upsets. She said food provided the only pleasure she currently had. I realized this was going to be challenging.

Suggested course of action

I felt we needed to go slowly in this instance. I gave the usual advice of not having anything in the house that she would be tempted to eat, such as the biscuits and cakes, and to only go shopping after a meal so she was less likely to add them to her trolley. I also suggested substituting her hot chocolate for one made with raw cacao powder, plant-based milk, a small amount of maple syrup and a spoonful of almond butter to make it satiating, and with considerably less sugar. I told her to have that first, and only after she had finished it could she eat anything else. I suggested this because I felt that once she was under the duvet (this was to be addressed at a later date), she wouldn't want to stir herself. We negotiated cutting down the takeaways to twice a week and trying to have two nights a week without alcohol. I hoped that these modest changes would make enough of a noticeable difference to spur her on to make some more. I kept the supplements to a multi vitamin and a probiotic, as well as vitamin D and *Crocus sativus* for her depression. Studies have shown that *Crocus sativus* is as effective as an antidepressant, without the side effects (see Chapter 9). The only other suggestion made at this stage was going for a walk with a friend who had kept asking how she could help. I explained how some gentle exercise (she wasn't doing any at this stage) and getting out in nature could help lift her mood a little.

Follow-up sessions

There wasn't huge progress regarding the dietary changes, so I decided to change tack and we focused the next session on her grief. As usual, I got her to tell her story, and there were, unsurprisingly, a lot of tears. It was encouraging to hear that she had a lot of support from both friends and her mum, but, so far, she seemed not to have accepted any of it and instead to have isolated herself. I asked if maybe her mum could take the kids occasionally so that she could perhaps book an aromatherapy session. It became clear that she was embarrassed about her size and having to take her clothes off, so we settled instead on reflexology, which she had had once before and had enjoyed. I gently prompted her about walking with her friend, and she said she would text her that evening. Having agreed to this self-care 'homework', I then suggested she read through my dietary advice from last time and commit to taking her supplements, reassuring her that they could make a significant difference to how she felt and the general state of her health. I felt it better not to push this, but she agreed she would try.

At the next session, Jenny told me she had been for a walk with her friend and that even though she had been reluctant, she had been glad that she did. She told me this friend was very supportive and wanted to be there for her and that the long walk had left her tired but in a good way. I asked if this could this be a regular thing, and she said her friend had suggested that they did it every Tuesday morning after dropping their kids off at school. I felt this was positive progress. Jenny had also had her reflexology session, which she found relaxing but had made her cry. The reflexologist had been very kind when Jenny told her she had lost her husband, and I let Jenny know that it was perfectly normal that this had prompted an emotional release and that this wasn't a bad thing. Jenny said she slept well that night and hadn't drunk any wine.

It seemed that focusing on self-care was a good way forward when working with Jenny, and my hope was that this would lead on to eventual changes to her diet. Our next couple of sessions were taken up with her expressing her grief, which continued to feel very necessary. When I asked if she still didn't want to live, she said she did still feel like that sometimes but not quite as strongly as before. We talked about how focusing on her children was helpful in keeping her here. I reinforced that there was no shame in feeling like this, that it was completely understandable, and she said that she appreciated being able to talk to someone who didn't judge her and that our sessions were helping her process what had happened.

Although sessions always remained firmly focused on Jenny, I decided it might be appropriate to share my own experience of grief so that Jenny would know I had personal understanding of the pain she was experiencing. I don't always do so, but sometimes it definitely helps to build rapport and lends a little additional weight to any suggestions I might give, when using myself as an example.

When I felt the time was right, I suggested we refocus on Jenny's diet, and she reluctantly agreed. She had actually managed to lose a little weight despite only making modest changes, but I offered praise for how well she'd done to achieve this. She'd originally said she'd like to get to a size-16 dress size by the summer, and I asked her how she felt about this goal now and whether it would be helpful to have something like this to focus on (i.e. trivial in comparison to her husband's death). She agreed that it might be and I emphasized how much better she might feel in terms of both health and self-esteem if she managed to work towards this goal.

I was taken by surprise at our next session when Jenny told me she had got a puppy. We had had a conversation about this in a previous session, discussing the pros and cons of getting a dog. I had mentioned that many bereaved people get pets, that a dog could be a really positive idea as you have to go out and walk it, regardless of how you feel, and that dogs can provide some much-needed affection after a loss. We also talked about how it would be great for the children. Although puppies can be hard work, Jenny had grown up with dogs, and I could see that this was definitely a positive decision for her. The additional exercise and being outside in the fresh air were clearly doing her good and the kids were delighted. We discussed using this as an impetus to really crack on with the dietary changes and cutting down on alcohol.

Jenny and I have gone on to work together for many months. Her diet improved further, and she has lost some more weight (though, as yet, not as much as she wants to). She only drinks wine at the weekends now and has cut back considerably on the takeaways, cakes and biscuits. She has more energy and the digestive upsets have disappeared. Her depression has lessened, she doesn't spend all day in bed any more, and now only occasionally does she feel that she doesn't want to live. We are currently talking about whether going back to work might be helpful or whether she's still not quite ready.

It would be misleading to neatly tie up this, or any other, account of a grieving client, by minimizing the still considerable and ongoing impact of the pain of grief that they all still feel to varying degrees. While I hope my support and advice helped to lessen their suffering in some way, I think it's necessary to emphasize that we are probably unlikely to see the transformation in health and wellbeing that we sometimes witness with our non-grieving clients. Nevertheless, walking with a grieving client and easing their path, in whatever small way might be possible, is a privilege.

These case studies don't cover every type of loss or demographic, but I hope they provide an insight into many of the losses that have far-reaching and long-lasting implications, such as loss of a parent at a young age, loss a partner, suicide and child loss.

CHAPTER 7

Platitudes

A common complaint made by bereaved people is how they feel their grief is often misunderstood or minimized. So, this chapter aims to offer a comprehensive understanding of what your grieving client is having to endure from those who proffer their unsolicited opinion. I hope that this will enable you as a practitioner, however well intentioned, to know what *not* to say, as well as gain some understanding of how thoughtless comments can impact your client's sense of wellbeing. As already mentioned, grieving clients usually feel extra sensitive and vulnerable, and need to be handled with particular care. It's important we try as much as we can to avoid saying anything that might inadvertently compound their pain.

A FEW PLATITUDES TO AVOID
'I know how you feel'

One of the temptations it is essential to resist, if you have experienced a loss yourself, is to say, 'I know how you feel.' It's understandable that you might say this as a way to establish rapport and show your empathy and compassion, but no two losses are the same. Anyway, this is about your client. You haven't experienced their grief and so you can't know exactly how it feels for them.

'Time heals all wounds'

It's true that for many things in life that cause us suffering, including some losses, the pain can lessen considerably with the passing of time. But most definitely not always. A grieving parent will never have the wound of losing their child completely healed by the passing of time, if at all. This may be the case for other losses too, so it's best to avoid this particular cliché. As bereaved father Bob Geldof said, 'Time doesn't heal, it accommodates',[1] which is a much more accurate and less offensive way of putting it.

'Everything happens for a reason'

You may think this is true and, in fact, even after my own experiences of losing both a child and a partner, I do, too. However, not everyone holds this belief. I would avoid saying this to anyone grieving because I have seen how offended people can be by this statement if it doesn't resonate with their beliefs. 'It was their time' is another pronouncement that some will take comfort from but others might take offence to, so best to err on the side of caution and avoid saying it.

'Lots of people go through difficult times'

This particular gem was said to me by a doctor. Yes, lots of people go through difficult times, but they are definitely not all of equal 'difficulty' and not all of them are traumatizing or life-changing. This minimizing and dismissal of someone's emotional pain (most especially from someone in the medical profession) is completely unacceptable.

---

1   Bob Geldof, as cited in Hayes, 2020

'At least they're no longer suffering'

This may well feel true to you, but how does this statement help the griever who is currently themselves suffering a great deal and would just rather have their person back? A lot of people feel very strongly when this dismissive remark is made to them. Also, avoid 'They had a good innings'. Even if someone lived a good and long life, this may not seem very relevant to a griever in the early days of loss.

'At least you have other children/can still have other children/can marry again'

I read of a bereaved mother who when told, 'At least you have other children', replied, 'Which one of *your* children could you do without?' This is such a good example of a well-intentioned attempt to make someone 'count their blessings' that is totally inappropriate given the gravity of their situation. As for still being able to have more children or get married again, even if this one day happens, the bereaved parent/widow/widower will still feel the loss of the child or partner who has died and remain deeply affected by their loss. And anyway, it definitely doesn't provide the intended comfort when the idea of having another child or finding another spouse is the very last thing they feel like thinking about in the depths of their grief. Basically, never start any sentence with 'At least'.

'Think positive'

Perhaps the most dismissive, insensitive and minimizing statement of them all. There are much better and more subtle ways of encouraging a grieving person on their path through grief. Also, 'You'll be all right'. This was said to me at my husband's funeral. I knew it was meant well, but it just felt like such a wildly inappropriate statement to make to a bereaved mother and widow just two weeks after her husband's death.

'What doesn't kill you makes you stronger'

Maybe some losses do make you stronger, but how can you know if theirs will? This may be intended to get them to look on the bright side, but this is unlikely to be apposite and is a grief- and trauma-avoidant cliché that will probably not land well.

'They'd want you to be happy/get on with your life'

Well, yes, but they'd also understand why the people they left behind are so heartbroken. This statement can instil a sense of failure and guilt for not doing better.

'God/the Universe doesn't give us more than we can handle'

Actually, he/it sometimes does, and that's why people take their own lives.

'You're so strong'

When in the presence of someone experiencing the depths of grief and trauma, it's best not to remind them of their perceived strength. I know it is meant to be a compliment and designed to encourage someone to keep going, but it's something that gets said a lot and, in my case, I found it left me feeling a sense of utter isolation. I felt that anyone who said this to me showed a lack of understanding that I had never felt less strong in my life. This felt so disappointing, because if they didn't understand that, how could they possibly support me?

'How did they die?'

The inappropriateness of this question has been mentioned earlier in the book but can bear further discussion in this section too, I think. I know that many of us have to enquire about family history and may need to know if there is a history of heart disease, cancer, etc. If the passing of a family member is not recent and/or they were elderly, then, handled with sensitivity, discussing this should not be too problematic. However, if someone is in early grief of any kind or has lost a close family member who died prematurely, then it's important to tread carefully. In these cases, asking how someone died can feel to the bereaved person like an extremely intrusive, not to mention dangerously triggering, question. What if the answer is murder or suicide? And even if it isn't, this question has the capacity to send someone right back to the actual passing and the emotional impact of the event. It's better to wait to be told. It's unbelievable how this is sometimes the first question someone will ask, particularly if it's a young person who has died. I would be completely put off by any wellness practitioner who asked this, rather than waiting for me to share – if I chose to.

TERMINOLOGY

This can be tricky – do you use 'died', 'passed over', 'passed away', 'crossed over'? I think, if possible, listen out for the terminology your client uses themselves and adopt that. If in doubt, you can always ask. Personally, I'd rather not have anyone walking on egg shells when it comes to this, and I will straightforwardly use the words 'died' and 'dead'. However, everyone is different, and I had a client who was extremely reactive to the word 'dead'. You may sometimes (though not always) find that the worse you consider the loss to be, the more your client may be brutally direct in certain ways, speaking very frankly and even being in possession of a very dark sense of humour. (This can probably be considered a trauma response, by the way.) However, a word of warning: while they may be shockingly direct, be mindful of not responding in kind. They are hurting, and if they've had experience of any of the insensitive remarks above, they may be all too ready to take offence. What's okay for them to say may not necessarily be okay for you to say.

Finally, a note on terminology used around suicide. You are most likely already aware that the term 'committed suicide' is to be avoided these days and rightly so. That term has the implication that someone who takes their own life has committed a crime or committed a sin, conveying shame and wrongdoing, harking back to days when suicide was indeed considered to be a crime or a sin. Hearing this outdated terminology could, as you can imagine, prove very upsetting to someone who has lost someone they love to suicide. Unfortunately, and rather shockingly, it's a term still being used by some, especially in some areas of the media. 'Died by suicide', 'took their own life' or 'ended their life' are terms usually considered more acceptable.

While the list of things to avoid saying may seem a bit daunting, no one is perfect and your client will no doubt understand if you make some small faux pas, especially if you apologize if you're worried you might have upset them. Here are a few ways you might find yourself on safer ground:

Mirror their reality

Rather than rushing to fix them or trying to 'bright side' them, agree that what they are going through is terrible. If they say the pain is like nothing they've ever experienced, reply that it must be. If things are dark, then allow them to be dark. Bear witness to their pain and acknowledge their reality. There may be no silver lining to be found in their situation, and even if there is, it's for them to discover. No toxic positivity!

Be with them where they are

If they want to talk about what happened, let them, rather than bringing them into the present and providing them with ways to make it better. Sometimes the healthiest thing a griever can do is simply sit with the pain of their loss and feel it. The only way out of the pain is through the pain and that has to happen in its own time. They are allowed to yearn for the person they have lost. Try to view the pain they feel as being proportionate to the love they feel – the deeper the love, the deeper the pain will probably be. Certainly, love can definitely exist alongside the pain. Bringing up the future and suggesting anything they could look forward to is sometimes best avoided when the loss has been great, because that's a place where the person who has died won't be and they may well still be adjusting to this. Let them be where they are. To try to move them on somewhere else could make them feel that where they are now is in some way wrong.

Trust them

They may be doing a lot to help themselves instinctively. Where you observe this, offer encouragement to follow their intuition. You may not know better than they do what's best for them right now. If you have some ideas about how you feel you can help, make a note of them and bring them up at a later session. However, if it feels right, you can always ask them how best you can support them, as opposed to deciding this for yourself.

Accept that it's their grief

Even if you think their grief is out of proportion to the situation or is going on too long in your view, don't minimize their feelings. It's their grief and needs to be respected. As Joanne Cacciatore, professor, grief counsellor and author, says, if you can't understand why someone is grieving so much, for so long, consider yourself fortunate that you don't understand.

Hold space for your grieving client

Pretty much the best approach that you can take, regardless of your modality, is to be willing to walk alongside your client without judging them, trying to fix them or attempting to affect any outcome. To reiterate, just offer unconditional support and try to let go of any need to attain results – this should be your priority with a grieving client. If we truly want to support someone through grief, we can't do it by taking their power away (trying to fix them), shaming them (implying that they should be doing better than they are) or overwhelming them (giving them more information than they're ready for). I know offering proactive advice is what many of us do – and this can undoubtedly contribute to their healing – but timing is everything. However, one message you can perhaps convey to them, when the time feels right, is that the pain they feel will change in time. They may not believe that it will improve, so 'change' is a better choice of word. It doesn't deny their pain but provides a realistic glimmer of hope that perhaps the intensity might shift.

I completely understand it can be so hard to let go of offering an opinion, trying to fix a client and make it better for them, but it is essential when working with a grieving client, at least initially, to resist this and to just hold space for them. This is particularly challenging for those of us who are nutritional therapists as we're so used to giving definitive advice. In coaching, on the other hand, our role is often to allow the client to work things through for themselves, giving them permission to trust their own intuition and wisdom, so this is perhaps a more appropriate approach in helping a grieving client to navigate their own unique path through grief. Empower them where possible to find their own answers, their own way forward, helping them to gain the resilience to keep going.

CHAPTER 8

Grief Models and Theories versus the Reality of Grief

The Five Stages of Grief Model

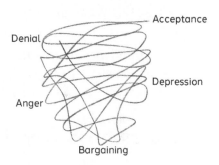

The Reality of Grief

It is to be hoped that we are starting to observe a sea change in grief awareness. As we know, not so long ago there was a lack of awareness and a stigma around mental health, and this has changed exponentially in the last few years. You could argue that even more people will be touched by grief than by mental health issues, as pretty much everyone will experience loss within their lifetime. Yet there remains a fear and stigma around death and grief, and sadly, for now, we still live in a grief-averse society.

As wellness practitioners, we can be at the forefront of this change if we educate ourselves about grief, especially as some areas of medicine and psychology are still often using outdated and unhelpful grief models. Some of our grieving clients, though by no means all of them, will be pretty clued up and well read on the subject of grief. I certainly was, so it jarred with me and created a disconnect when I came across a professional of any kind who wasn't. As we know, doctors have woefully little training in the importance that nutrition can play in the health of their patients (generally, around 10–24 hours over five to six years in medical school is spent on nutrition), and I've heard there is a comparable issue with psychologists and psychotherapists and the time given to grief in their training...

Most of us probably aren't doctors, psychologists or psychothera-pists, but we can provide credible support for grievers in all manner of ways, as we have already explored, especially if we educate ourselves on the reality of grief and keep up to date on the latest research – in the way that we do for other aspects of our work. If we can demon-strate knowledge, responsibility and professionalism, then this will instil confidence in our clients that we properly understand grief and that we therefore have the capability to help them effectively.

KÜBLER-ROSS'S FIVE STAGES OF GRIEF

There are several 'grief models', and some of them are discussed below, but the most famous grief model of them all is the 'five stages of grief' which, although now challenged, is still being used very literally by some psychologists, therapists and bereavement coun-sellors today. It was developed by Elisabeth Kübler-Ross and became famous after she published her book *On Death and Dying* in 1969.[1] In fact, this 'grief model' wasn't developed for grievers at all but was used by Kübler-Ross to describe people with terminal illness facing their own death. However, it was then adapted as a road map for the grieving process and has been interpreted as a way to somehow strategize grief and reduce it to five easy steps, despite the fact that

---

1   Kübler-Ross, 2014

no study has ever established that the five stages of grief actually exist. It is misleading to promote the idea that there is an orderly and predictable pattern that everyone will go through, implying that if you don't successfully get through the stages, you might remain stuck in the pain of grief for ever.

The main confusion around the five stages of grief is that they are believed by many to be linear and that somehow once you reach the 'goal' of acceptance, then well done, you've completed your grief journey. It's now generally agreed that you can't, and shouldn't, try to package grief with all its very messy emotions into a neat 'one size fits all' formula. In fact, Kübler-Ross, in her writing, makes it clear that the stages are non-linear, that people can experience these aspects of grief at different times and they do not happen in a certain order. Unfortunately, her intention somehow got lost along the way and the model became implemented very literally.

As you will see below, as emotions in their own right, denial, anger, bargaining, depression and acceptance make sense as part of a complex maelstrom of emotions that might be felt during the grieving process. However, some people might not experience all of the five stages, and some might find their feelings vary with different bereavements. Many would argue that several more stages could be added in, that grief goes back and forth through the stages, that denial, anger, bargaining and depression may be experienced many, many times, and that sometimes acceptance is never reached at all – and even if it is, the previous stages can still be experienced all over again. Unfortunately, the adoption of this model of grief has left some grievers (and sometimes their therapists and counsellors) with the expectation that once the stages have been gone through in a particular order, the grief will be done with. This can be harmful, leading to a feeling of not getting grief right, which is fundamentally very unhelpful because there is really no right or wrong way to do grief.

So, these five stages of grief have become ingrained in our cultural consciousness despite the fact that the model really doesn't accurately describe most people's experiences of grief – unsurprising perhaps when Kübler-Ross didn't develop it as a model for the bereaved and apparently regretted that it became so misunderstood. As you will see below, the issue really isn't that a bereaved person will or won't potentially experience these *feelings*; it's more to do with the idea that there are steps to be got through and in a specific order so that grief can be 'completed'. To reiterate, the stages won't necessarily be in this order, they may be experienced many times, there will be many other emotions in addition, and reaching some kind of acceptance doesn't necessarily mean the grieving process is over.

Denial

Denial can undoubtedly serve an important purpose. When life suddenly makes no sense after a loss and someone is in a state of shock, denial can be protective, helping a griever pace out their feelings and allowing them to begin to adapt to their new situation. Feeling numb in the early days of bereavement can be very common, and some people may appear to carry on as if nothing has happened. Denial and shock help them to cope, making survival possible. It's as if it's nature's way of letting in only as much as a bereaved person can handle. Even if they know with their heads that someone has died, it can still be hard to properly grasp that they're not coming back. As they gradually begin to accept the reality of the loss, any feelings they were denying may begin to surface.

Anger

Anger is very natural after someone dies. Death can seem cruel and unfair, especially when someone has suffered or has died 'before their time', and this can therefore most definitely lead to feelings of anger. It's also common to feel angry towards the person who has died, or angry at ourselves for things we did or didn't do before their death. The more the anger is allowed to be felt, the more it will begin to dissipate. Underneath that anger is pain. Grief expert David Kessler says:

It is natural to feel deserted and abandoned, but we live in a society that fears anger. Anger is strength and it can be an anchor, giving temporary structure to the nothingness of loss. At first grief feels like being lost at sea: no connection to anything. Then you get angry at someone, maybe a person who didn't attend the funeral, maybe a person who isn't around, maybe a person who is different now that your loved one has died. Suddenly you have a structure – your anger toward them. The anger becomes a bridge over the open sea, a connection from you to them. It is something to hold on to; and a connection made from the strength of anger feels better than nothing.[2]

Bargaining

When someone we love has died, it can feel hard to accept that there's nothing we can do to change things. Bargaining is when we start to make deals with ourselves, or perhaps with God. We want to believe that if we act in a certain way, we will feel better. It's very common to find ourselves going over things that happened in the past and asking 'what if' and 'if only'. We would give anything to go back and change things in the hope everything could have turned out differently. We want life to go back to how it was, and we desperately want our loved one with us again. 'Magical thinking' – the belief that our thoughts, actions, words can influence the course of events – may be experienced. Guilt is often a companion of bargaining because the 'if onlys' can lead to us blaming ourselves and what we think we should have done differently. We may bargain with the grief and feel we will do anything not to feel the pain of this loss. Bargaining is about trying to somehow negotiate our way out of the hurt.

Depression

Sooner or later, and often many times over, the intense sadness of grief will deepen. Life can feel as if it no longer holds any meaning,

---

2   'The Five Stages of Grief™: Anger' in Kessler, n.d.

which can be very frightening. Nevertheless, depression is the appropriate response to a great loss, even though it feels as though it will last forever. Kessler says:

> We withdraw from life, left in a fog of intense sadness, wondering, perhaps, if there is any point in going on alone? Why go on at all? Depression after a loss is too often seen as unnatural: a state to be fixed, something to snap out of. The first question to ask yourself is whether or not the situation you're in is actually depressing. The loss of a loved one is a very depressing situation, and depression is a normal and appropriate response. To not experience depression after a loved one dies would be unusual.[3]

Acceptance

This is probably the most controversial stage. Perhaps, rather than seeing it as the 'completion' stage to be achieved so that we no longer grieve or miss our loved one, we instead need to see it as accepting the reality that our loved one is physically gone and recognizing that this new reality is permanent. Depending on the loss, some people may never fully get over the death of a loved one, but most will eventually accept that living without them is their new reality. This doesn't mean that they're okay with what's happened, just that they now accept they can't change the situation and that they have to find a way to learn to live with it. Difficult though it undoubtedly is, life without the loved one has to be adjusted to. This 'acceptance' of the situation doesn't, however, mean that denial, anger, bargaining and depression won't be felt again.

The sixth stage of grief – finding meaning

In 2019, David Kessler (who co-authored *On Grief and Grieving* with Elizabeth Kübler-Ross) wrote his book *Finding Meaning: The Sixth*

---

3   'The Five Stages of Grief™: Depression' in Kessler, n.d.

Stage of Grief.[4] Despite his respected expertise, stemming from years of working as a grief expert, his life was devasted beyond anything he could previously imagine by the sudden death of his 21-year-old son. He knew he had to find a path through this terrible loss and a way that would honour his son, so he added a sixth stage of grief: meaning. He argues that rather than looking for closure, finding meaning can transform grief into a more peaceful and hopeful experience. We will look at ways your client might find some kind of meaning after their loss and explore the concept of post-traumatic growth in Chapter 10. Details of *Finding Meaning* and other books on grief that might be useful to recommend to your grieving client can also be found in Chapter 10.

Emotions you might observe in your client that are not covered by the five stages model

Your client may experience so many other emotions besides denial, anger, bargaining and depression. They may express to you that they feel numbness, fear, regret, yearning, relief, resentment, shame, overwhelm or guilt, for example. Guilt is extremely common because it's often easier to feel guilty than it is to feel helpless. Guilt and blaming themselves is somehow preferable to feeling that they have no power at all, no control over their loved one's death. It's important to remember that some of the thoughts and feelings experienced in grief are not necessarily logical but occur because the mind just desperately wants to try and make some kind of sense of what has happened.

BOWLBY'S STAGES OF GRIEF

John Bowlby was a well-known British psychologist and psychiatrist who was a pioneer of attachment theory in children and wrote a trilogy of books called *Attachment and Loss.*[5] He took all his observations

---

4   Kessler, 2019
5   Bowlby, 1997

and theories about attachment and separation and applied them to grief and bereavement. He believed that a response to grief was based on the environment and the psychological makeup of the griever. As a bereaved mother and widow, I would argue that these are only part of what informs a response to grief. I don't believe the intense grief felt in child loss, for example, can be defined quite so reductively. Bowlby believed that the 'affectional bond', as he referred to it, is broken by death, and it is this that results in grief. He divided grief into four stages, which are generally less well known than those of Kübler-Ross. Similarly, they have some merit but are again flawed as a 'one size fits all' model of grief.

Shock and numbness

This is the stage where there is a sense that the loss is not real and appears impossible to accept. Bowlby acknowledged that there can be physical distress during this phase. He believed that if someone did not progress well through this phase, they would struggle to accept and understand or communicate their emotions.

Yearning and searching

During this stage, there is a preoccupation with the person who has died and a constant yearning and searching for reminders of them and ways to be close to them. If we cannot progress through this phase, Bowlby believed, then we will spend our life trying to fill the void of the loss and remain preoccupied with the person who had died.

Despair and disorganization

In this stage, there is an acceptance that everything has changed and will not go back to the way it was. As a result, there is a sense of hopelessness and despair, as well as anger and questioning. There may also be a withdrawal from others. Bowlby thought that if we don't progress through this phase, we will remain consumed by anger and depression, and that our attitude towards life will remain negative and hopeless. He believed, however, that anger is necessary for a healthy outcome in grieving.

Reorganization and recovery

Eventually, faith in life starts to become restored. The griever starts to rebuild their life, establishing new patterns and goals, and trust in life is slowly restored. In this phase, the grief does not go away, nor is it fully resolved, but, according to Bowlby, the loss recedes and shifts to a hidden section of the brain, where it continues to influence us but is no longer at the forefront of the mind.

MEANING-CENTRED PROCESS MODEL

Paul Wong's grief model involves four main processes that follow individual paths of recovery, all of which may interact with each other.[6] With this particular grief model, the emphasis is on transformation through meaning. The first process is mourning the loss, which Wong believes begins with numbness and shock, before moving on to the turbulence of more intense emotions (including anger, guilt, shame, regret, etc.) and leading eventually to the calmer state of sadness. He acknowledges that this process is not linear but that the feelings involved may become less intense and less frequent and can be interspersed with more positive emotions. In his view, sifting through, and adjusting to, the conflicting emotions of grief contributes to recovery.

The second path is accepting the loss, which involves the complicated process of acknowledging its finality in multiple ways, on a cognitive, social, behavioural, existential, spiritual and emotional level. He believes the last of these may be the most difficult task when the emotional attachment is strong but that acceptance on an emotional level is necessary in order to be able to 'let go'. The third task

6   Wong, 2008

is adjusting to the loss. This entails adapting to new dynamics within both the family and a wider social structure. This stage may also involve working on both the self and relationships, and could include dealing with issues such as forgiveness and conflict resolution.

Wong's fourth process is about transforming the loss. This, he believes, is essential to recovery. In his view, the loss has to become incorporated into the present and the future. This happens by moving from the initial struggles of the grieving process and on to a restructured existence where the griever begins to establish new life goals, new plans for their future and a redefining of their identity. It's about finding new meaning in life and a different perspective on the loss, the past and the future. Wong says that he considers this transformation necessary for resolving grief and also for personal growth. However, he believes it would be difficult to experience the transformation without adopting the attitude of approach acceptance (which implies belief in a happy afterlife; individuals who believe in an afterlife are more likely to show less fear of death) or neutral acceptance (in which death is considered an integral part of life; to be alive is to live with death and dying, neither fearing or welcoming it), as described in detail in the Death Attitude Profile.[7]

I quite like some aspects of this model, including Wong's acknowledgement of spiritual acceptance as part of the grieving process and that this may involve establishing a spiritual connection with the deceased. However, I have an issue with his use of the words 'recovery' (grief is not an illness) and 'resolution' (as Megan Devine would say, grief is not a problem that needs to be resolved). His view that the griever can let go of their grief (and perhaps by implication their loved one) once they have achieved acceptance at the emotional level is in contrast to the continuing bonds theory which maintains there is no need to 'let go'. I suspect many who have experienced a significant loss are going to struggle with certain elements of these stages from Paul Wong.

---

7   Gesser, Wong and Reker, 1988; Wong, Reker and Gesser, 1994.

WORDEN'S FOUR TASKS FOR MOURNING

Yet another grief model was devised by psychologist J. William Worden,[8] who provides a framework of four tasks for the bereaved. He advocates that healing happens gradually as grievers address these tasks, acknowledging, thankfully, that this happens in no specific order, and that you may go back and forth from one to another over time – so at least some progress from the (perceived) linear models. I do have a slight issue with the word 'task', which rather gives the impression of a 'to do' list or checking off a few DIY jobs. A task is not really a word I would associate with going through the pain of grief.

As there is some overlap with previous models, the summary here is brief:

Task 1: To accept the reality of the loss
This refers to integrating the reality of the death over time.

Task 2: To process the pain of grief
Grief needs to be processed emotionally, cognitively, physically and spiritually.

Task 3: To adjust to a world without the deceased
External adjustments include taking on responsibilities and learning new skills. Internal adjustments are made as the griever adapts to their new identity. Spiritual adjustments occur as they are challenged about their belief system and the purpose and meaning of life.

8   Worden, 2009

Task 4: To find an enduring connection with the deceased in the midst of embarking on a new life

Working towards finding a balance between continuing to remember the person who died and living a full and meaningful life.

Worden believes mourning is successfully concluded when all four tasks are completed. Again, these models are all very well in theory, but in practice it feels a bit like a test, with the pressure that comes with it. Fine if you're an academic, less so if you're grieving a significant loss.

Next, we come to the grief model that is by far the best, in my view.

TONKIN'S MODEL OF GRIEF

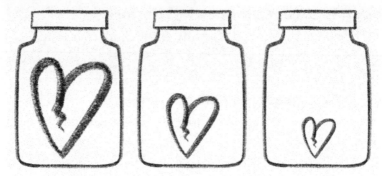

It's often assumed that grief lessens with time.

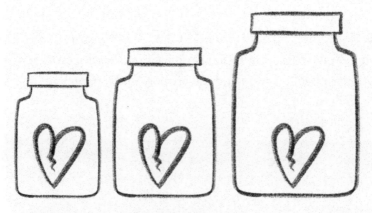

In reality, grief stays the same but gradually life grows around it.

This model of grief is altogether simpler. It is, in my view, the best of all of those outlined in this chapter. The 'growing around grief' model was created by grief counsellor Lois Tonkin,[9] which she devised after she spoke to a client about the death of her child. The bereaved mother told Tonkin that, to begin with, grief filled every part of her life and was all-consuming. She drew a picture with a circle to represent her life and shading to indicate her grief. She had thought that, as time went by, the grief would shrink and become a much smaller part of her life. But, in fact, the grief stayed just as big, but her life grew around it. There were times where she felt the grief as intensely as when her child first died, but then, eventually, there were other times when she felt she lived her life in the space outside the circle (or heart in the illustration) of her grief.

Tonkin's 'growing around grief' model demonstrates how we can still grieve the loss of our loved one, but we can also – at the same time – grow a new life which *includes* the loss. It suggests that, over time, your grief may stay much the same, but your life will begin to grow around it. This model of grief feels far less pressurized than the race of the five stages model or some of the other challenging and exacting models. Personally speaking, it feels a relief, with Tonkin's model, not to be told that the grief will go away in time if I can somehow accomplish the completion of certain 'stages' or 'tasks', because that simply doesn't feel possible or achievable to me or, I expect, to many others. Instead, Tonkin's model acknowledges that there will be some days where you feel grief as strongly as you did when the person first died, but there will eventually also be days when you are able to get on with, and even enjoy, other aspects of your life. So, the 'growing around grief' model shows how we can integrate our loss into the life we now lead. We will still grieve the loss of our loved one, while living our lives to the best of our ability. It shows that we can grow a new life around, and *including*, our loss, and that is far

---

9   Tonkin, 1996

more comforting and attainable for many grieving people. This is the grief model I suggest you might want to share with your clients.

The reality is that grief looks different for everyone and some losses are going to be more challenging than others. Perhaps rather than looking to the Kübler-Ross or the other models, or indeed any other way of sanitizing the inconveniently messy business of grief, it might be preferable to encourage your client to just go with the flow of grief, without any requirement to have to identify any particular 'stage' or emotion. Perhaps, instead, it's healthier to trust that the soul/mind/body knows how to process grief, if allowed to do so without interference. I prefer to look at grief from the point of view of ongoing healing and to allow it to free-flow, shape-shifting as it goes. Healing in grief is, in my view, about living *despite* the pain of loss, not with the end goal of somehow mastering it, as appears to be the perceived expectation of some of the grief models. The author Tom Zuba (who lost two children and his wife) says that when it comes to grief, healing from loss isn't a destination but rather an ongoing process. He says, 'Healing now becomes my way of being in the world.'[10] When someone has experienced a profound loss or losses, this is both an encouraging and realistic hypothesis. Perhaps this might be an altogether better and gentler concept to convey to our grieving clients.

The purpose of outlining these models is so that you are not only well informed if you have a client who asks you about them, but so you can be discerning about how realistic they are for something as complex and varied as grief. One of the questions I ask my clients – for just about anything during the grieving process frankly – is 'Does it help or does it hinder?' Grief is hard enough to go through as it is, without imposing unhelpful 'rules' for how to do it. Some of your clients will be resourceful at finding their own path through grief, and finding you might be one way they're doing so, but what if they feel they need (or it's been suggested by their friends or family) more

10 Zuba, 2018, p.1

traditional ways of getting through grief in addition to your support? Getting on the waiting list for bereavement counselling and taking antidepressants prescribed after a visit to the GP seem to be the most typical courses of action for acquiring help after a loss.

My observation is that grieving clients start off very keen to get some sort of counselling or therapy (and this was also true in my own case) but can often find it disappointing in reality. This won't always be the case, however, and some will be fortunate to find the help they're looking for from bereavement counselling or therapy. But how do you advise them on this subject, if asked for your opinion?

SHOULD YOU RECOMMEND SEEKING THE HELP OF A BEREAVEMENT THERAPIST OR COUNSELLOR?

Having read this far (and with more advice and tools to come), you will be starting to feel more comfortable and confident in supporting your grieving client, but what if you feel they still need something you don't feel able to provide? Should you recommend they see a bereavement counsellor or a therapist? It depends. If you know of someone who specializes in grief, and you definitely know that they're good, then, yes, of course. But just vaguely saying to your grieving client, 'Why don't you look for a bereavement counsellor?' is a slightly different matter. Because it can be a minefield. Finding the right therapist is hard enough in ordinary life, but for your grieving client, with possible fatigue and brain fog, searching for someone who will be a good fit can be overwhelming. I know because I tried.

I ought to disclose here that, after my son died, I did not find the support I needed from grief and trauma therapists or bereavement counsellors, and eventually I gave up. My experience was that I felt no one really properly got the reality of my grief, that in many ways I knew more than they did about loss, especially the particular magnitude of child loss. Sadly, I know many bereaved parents who have shared my experience but, in fairness, I also know that some did manage to find a good therapist who offered the support they were looking for.

It may be your client is on a long waiting list to see a bereavement counsellor and has come to you in the meantime to support them through a different approach. They may still feel they need the support they think a counsellor can provide and ask specifically if you can recommend anyone. If you don't know a therapist who works specifically with grief, you could perhaps offer the following advice to your client as a starting point. First, following on from this chapter and previous ones, suggest they watch out for language that suggests grief is a problem that can be fixed, for any toxic positivity, talk of 'recovery' or any mention of the dreaded five stages. Any of the above may indicate a belief that grief somehow needs correction and potentially demonstrates that grief is not their strong point and that they may not be up to date with the latest reading and research in this area.

Many therapists will list grief as one of a great number of areas they work in. For instance, if you put 'grief' into the search bar of a therapist directory, you will see just how many therapists list grief as a so-called 'specialism' – along with many other areas of expertise. It's rather like, as nutritional therapists, before we were all encouraged to niche, we all probably listed IBS, for example. Some of us will be more expert in this area than others – but if we all say that we are, how is a potential client really meant to identify a true specialism and the expertise they require? We can apply this same premise to therapists and grief – and many of them probably have far less training in grief than nutritional therapists have in IBS, as we will see below.

Although this section is not focused on instances where you feel there is a serious mental health issue (in which case you must, of course, refer on), you might want to suggest to your client that they look for a therapist who describes themselves as 'trauma-informed' if it's relevant to them and their experience of loss. As previously discussed, EMDR and CBT are forms of therapy often recommended for trauma and PTSD, so you could suggest your client looks into this to see if these are therapies that they feel might suit them, and they can then look specifically for therapists who specialize in them. Maybe also suggest that your client really thinks about what it is they want from therapy or counselling. This may help them to focus, as well as manage their expectations if they are secretly hoping there is someone out there who might hold a magic key to making it all better. Unfortunately, no one is that good.

As you will have learned by now, everyone's experience of grief is very different, so not all of your clients will need counselling or therapy for their grief. A common experience many of us have when first bereaved is to be asked by those around us if we're going to get bereavement counselling, so it's possible some of your clients might feel it's an expectation of something they 'should' do. Some of them, though, will find they actually have sufficient resilience to cope with their loss, especially if they are fortunate to have your support. However, this might not always be enough if the grief was traumatic. It's also worth bearing in mind that, in the coming years, it's thought that a greater number of people than usual are likely to seek extra help due to the loss of a loved one during the pandemic, whether because of Covid directly, or another cause of death during that time. The issues caused by the restrictions, such as not being able to say goodbye or hold a proper funeral, may have complicated the grieving process and therefore an increasing number of people may seek bereavement support.

According to an article by Katherine King entitled 'Grief and loss: Will therapists be able to help?' in *Psychology Today*, the next pandemic will be one of grief, and many therapists are not equipped for this possibility because, King believes, the subject of death and grief has been neglected for far too long: 'Within programs that train therapists, the required coursework on these topics is paltry at best. Students frequently graduate having had only brief exposure to the topic and no formal training on effective clinical interventions.'[11]

---

11 King, 2020

A recent study found that almost 46 per cent of clients did not find their mental health professional helpful during their grief.[12] The article by King goes on to say that most therapists in practice today have insufficient preparation for the coming tidal wave of grieving clients and that those with more complicated grief may even be harmed by under-prepared clinicians.[13] Another study interviewed people who had received grief support and found many left feeling 'frustrated, confused, abandoned, and overwhelmed at a particularly vulnerable time'.[14]

King believes that therapists must be trained better in grief and death in order to improve current standards. She believes they aren't properly educated about the research on what actually helps different types of grieving clients, and so consequently are unable to make appropriate suggestions. She points out that clients assume that a professionally qualified therapist will have the expertise to help them and that, in this, they may be mistaken. (As I say, this has been my observation, too.) It's really quite concerning and not something our clients would probably ever imagine to be the case when they are seeking a grief therapist in all good faith. They assume training and expertise, specifically in grief, will be a given.

I believe that there are, of course, really good therapists and counsellors out there who can help with grief, but I also think the reality is there are many who, for whatever reason, will sadly make no discernible difference to your client. While I'm not suggesting you discourage them from trying to find someone, it may be worth pointing out that finding a therapist or counsellor with the expertise they need for their grief might not be quite as easy as they think. Arguably, this is no different for people seeking our services as wellness practitioners. However, potential clients are quite possibly more discerning about checking our qualifications, testimonials and experience as 'alternative' therapists than they are for 'mainstream'

---

12   Aoun *et al.*, 2019
13   King, 2020
14   Valentine, McKell and Ford, 2017

therapists and counsellors, who they assume are experienced in the areas they say they specialize in and therefore will be able to help them effectively. A client who is grieving can be especially vulnerable, and that can lead to disappointment if their expectations are not met.

Megan Devine, a psychotherapist herself, makes the following wise observation which can be applied to therapists and wellness practitioners alike: 'What you need are those things – those people, those places, those words – that come up underneath you and give you roots. You need those things that nourish you, that help you do the work your heart is already doing.'[15]

The reality of grief is that there is no panacea, no magic formula and no one practitioner or therapist who can 'solve' or 'fix' grief. Some losses are harder to bear, and it will probably be the clients who have experienced those who may be looking for anything – and any-one – who might ease their suffering. However, don't underestimate how important your own expertise and support can be in helping them in their healing and, as Devine says, giving them roots and helping them do the work that their heart has to do when grieving.

There are also resources you can suggest to your client in the Appendix, such as support groups, which can be particularly useful for bereaved parents and widows/widowers. Grief can be an isolating experience, so the importance of talking to, or working with, some-one who walks in your shoes cannot be underestimated – which is why I now support clients through my own method of grief support.[16] The purpose of this section has been to provide context around the reality of grief counselling and therapy being assumed to be the gold standard for helping someone who is bereaved. It can be, of course, with the right therapist, but there are other often equally valid ways your grieving client can be supported through their grief – and some of these ways can be provided by you.

_____

15   Devine, 2014
16   www.wellbeingandnutrition.co.uk

CHAPTER 9

Nutritional Medicine Support

Every grieving client is unique in their circumstances, personality, mindset and symptoms, and, most importantly, unique in their experience of grief. Therefore, much of the following nutritional medicine advice has to be general. Then, of course, there is the question of contraindications between medication and supplements, which means any suggestions here can only act as a guide. If you are a nutritional therapist or naturopath, you will have your own way of supporting your clients through dietary and lifestyle changes and the use of targeted supplements. If you practise something else, it may not be in your remit to be able to recommend specific supplements, though you may still find some of this chapter of interest.

Understanding how grief and trauma can interrupt the bidirectional communication between the brain and the body can help you to get to the root of your client's issues, rather than just treating the physical symptoms in themselves. Separating the brain and body, as many of us are aware, misses the bigger picture. We need to support our grieving clients both psychologically and physically, invariably paying particular attention to regulating their nervous system. We can do this through coaching, breathwork, yoga, reiki and a myriad of other modalities that can help them to sleep better, feel less fatigued and anxious, reduce inflammation and improve gut health.

Without doubt, nutritional therapy has a big contribution to make to all of these issues.

As you will see from the case studies in Chapter 6, a probiotic and a good-quality multi vitamin and mineral will probably form the basis of any supplement programme, just as it might for any of your clients. However, an alternative approach would be to use, either instead or in addition, individual nutrients or a supplement complex designed to support the nervous system. You may also want to look at digestive, adrenal-, hormonal- or immune-supportive supplements, where appropriate, as well as dietary measures. Then you may decide to add something for sleep or mood if this is a particular issue. Obviously, if your client has booked a package of sessions with you, this can be built on over time. If you're not a registered nutritional therapist or naturopath and you feel some of these suggestions might be of help to your client, then please recommend they seek the help of a BANT-registered nutritional therapist.

THE GUT AND GRIEF

As with every client we see, the state of their microbiome is crucial to their overall health. We know their gut health can be affected by poor diet, stress and lifestyle factors, which can result in a reduction in the abundance of bacterial species in the gut. In the case of a grieving client, especially one with anxiety or PTSD, the gut–brain axis, which links the emotional and cognitive centres of the brain with peripheral intestinal functions, can become adversely affected. As we saw with Andrew in Chapter 6, his grief and trauma directly impacted the functioning of his gut. Some of the symptoms seen during the initial stages of grief are discussed in Chapter 3. Many of these symptoms, as we can see, are gut-related – for example, nausea, loss of appetite, a speeded-up metabolism, digestive upset, increase or decrease in appetite and a hollow feeling in stomach.

The vagus nerve

The connection between the gut and the nervous system is unbreakable, and it is the vagus nerve that creates this two-way communication path. The vagus nerve is the longest of the nerves that arise from the brain, and it communicates with different parts of the body, modulating several essential processes. It is a key part of the parasympathetic 'rest and digest' nervous system and counterbalances the sympathetic nervous system's fight-or-flight mechanism. It influences breathing, digestive function and heart rate, all of which can have a huge impact on mental health. Unfortunately, chronic and traumatic stress interrupts this bidirectional communication between the brain and the body, affecting the vagal brake and its ability to calm and regulate the nervous system. The sensitive vagus nerve picks up information from the body (e.g. from the lungs, liver, intestines and heart) and sends it to the brain for analysis and interpretation. The brain then sends messages and commands back down to the organs.

Vagal tone reflects the ratio between sympathetic and parasympathetic signals. A low vagal tone means the vagus nerve isn't functioning as it should, potentially resulting in depression, anxiety, gut issues and inflammation. Increasing your vagal tone activates the parasympathetic nervous system, and having higher vagal tone means that your body can relax faster after stress. It reduces heart rate and blood pressure, changes the function of certain parts of the brain and encourages healthy digestion. By stimulating the vagus nerve, we are able to send a message to the body to relax and de-stress, leading to improvements in mood, wellbeing and resilience. The advice for healing and revitalizing healthy function of the vagus nerve usually centres around supporting gut health through diet and probiotics, breathing techniques, meditation, cold showers or splashing the face with cold water, foot massage, exercise and connecting with nature.

There are very few studies to date that have investigated how stress may lead to changes in the gut microbiota in the context of bereavement, and much of that research is only from animal model studies. A 2020 study concluded that '[u]ltimately, it is possible that stress may change microbiota and vice versa via neuroendocrine, inflammatory, and behavioral (e.g., depression) pathways, but additional research is needed on this topic in general and especially in the context of bereavement'.[1] Nevertheless, we can work on the hypothesis that grief is a major stress event and that because it's established that stress can alter the state of the microbiome and in turn can increase the level of colonic inflammation, it is very likely that the gut is going to be affected during grief. However, the extent of this will be determined by the unique profile of your client.

There is no doubt that alongside looking at eliminating foods that might typically exacerbate any digestive symptoms (such as wheat, sugar and dairy), the inclusion of gut-supportive foods and supplements is going to provide a good foundation for most grieving clients. Fermented foods such as kefir, yogurt with live active cultures, pickled vegetables, tempeh, kombucha tea, kimchi, miso and sauerkraut can be suggested, if appropriate. In addition to a probiotic supplement, and depending on the symptoms your client might be experiencing, aloe vera, digestive enzymes, L-glutamine, marshmallow and slippery elm may also be worth considering. Many of the supplement companies combine some of these ingredients into one supplement.

Serotonin, mood and the gut

Mood-boosting serotonin is a neurotransmitter that helps to send messages from one area of the brain to another. It is believed that serotonin is linked to brain cells involved in a range of psychological processes, as well as brain cells that influence some body functions and systems. It is estimated that gut bacteria manufacture around 90 per cent of the body's supply of serotonin. Chronic stress is a known cause of low serotonin and so a depletion of serotonin is quite

---

1   Seiler, von Känel and Slavich, 2020

likely to be found during bereavement. Establishing a healthy diversity of gut flora is therefore something of a priority for ensuring the production if serotonin. As we know, the gut–brain axis is a bidirectional communication system between the central nervous system and the gastrointestinal tract, and this was highlighted by a study titled 'Serotonin, tryptophan metabolism and the brain-gut-microbiome axis':

> Serotonin functions as a key neurotransmitter at both terminals of this network. In particular, it is becoming clear that the microbial influence on tryptophan metabolism and the serotonergic system may be an important node in such regulation. There is also substantial overlap between behaviours influenced by the gut microbiota and those which rely on intact serotonergic neurotransmission. The enzymes of this pathway are immune and stress-responsive, both systems which buttress the brain–gut axis. In addition, there are neural processes in the gastrointestinal tract which can be influenced by local alterations in serotonin concentrations with subsequent relay of signals along the scaffolding of the brain–gut axis to influence CNS neurotransmission. Therapeutic targeting of the gut microbiota might be a viable treatment strategy for serotonin-related brain–gut axis disorders.[2]

Aside from the inclusion of probiotic food and supplements, another way to raise serotonin is meditation, which is believed to increase serotonin because it relieves stress. Fresh air and sunlight also improve mood and serotonin levels, as can exercise. Therefore, a multifaceted approach is, as always, a good idea.

---

2   O'Mahony *et al.*, 2015, p.32

Foods that might help to raise serotonin levels

The amino acid tryptophan is a precursor to serotonin, so eating foods containing tryptophan may help the body produce more serotonin and therefore enhance mood. Eggs, spinach, salmon, tofu, nuts, seeds, turkey and any foods high in protein, iron, vitamins B2 and B6 all tend to contain good levels of tryptophan. While foods high in this amino acid won't necessarily boost serotonin on their own, they may when in combination with complex carbohydrates. Carbohydrates cause the body to release more insulin, which promotes amino acid absorption. Therefore, if you mix high-tryptophan foods with complex carbohydrates, you might get a serotonin boost.

THE IMPORTANCE OF BLOOD SUGAR BALANCE DURING GRIEF

As we know, trauma in grief can trigger an increase in the body's fight-or-flight hormone, cortisol, due to the assumption that's it's under attack. In response to this, the body releases extra energy into the bloodstream in the form of glucose to give you the necessary fuel to fight or flee. When chronically heightened, cortisol works against glucose control, even in people who don't have diabetes, so it's not difficult to see how this can become an issue if the stress of grief continues long-term.

Unfortunately, type 2 diabetes is a condition that can sometimes be associated with bereavement. A growing body of research indicates that stress plays a role, both as a predictor of new-onset type 2 diabetes and as a prognostic factor for individuals with existing type 2 diabetes. Stress-related biological pathways that are believed to contribute include chronic activation of the hypothalamic pituitary adrenal (HPA) axis, leading to dysregulated cortisol output that can then give rise to glucose intolerance and systemic insulin resistance. (For those who might not know, the HPA axis is the central stress response system. It's required for stress adaptation. Activation of the HPA axis causes secretion of glucocorticoids, which act on multiple organ systems to redirect energy resources to meet real or anticipated demand. HPA axis dysfunction refers to how chronic stress breaks down the very system in the body needed for a healthy stress response.)

How to advise your grieving client on keeping blood sugar balanced

It will probably be obvious to many of you to recommend regular meals with a good level of protein and some healthy fats and to avoid sugary foods and refined carbohydrates, in order to keep blood sugar on an even keel. It's important not to avoid all carbohydrates, though, as if you recommend cutting them out during the stress of grief, it may reinforce the body's belief that it's in survival mode and it might then increase cortisol in order to deal with this. So, there is definitely a place for some complex carbohydrates in the diet, such as pulses, brown rice, oats and quinoa, along with a good variety of vegetables.

Always bear in mind that if your client is in early grief, they may struggle to follow much of your guidance, so you may need to simplify your advice in order of importance, based on their particular needs. Prioritizing the avoidance of high glycaemic index (GI) foods (cakes, sweets, white bread, etc.) may need to take precedence because of their enhanced ability to increase blood glucose, with the potential to accelerate a compensatory insulin release leading to a blood sugar crash (reactive hypoglycaemia). Hypoglycaemia is associated with an increase in the stress hormones adrenaline and cortisol, which is most definitely unwanted.

Encouraging you client to eat a low-GI diet to help with balancing blood sugar might include the following recommendations:

- 5–7 portions of vegetables each day and 1–2 portions of berries or apple
- protein at every meal – meat, fish, eggs or plant-based (organic tofu, tempeh, beans, lentils, chickpeas)

- complex carbohydrates – quinoa, brown rice, wild rice, sweet potatoes, lentils or soba noodles
- fats – oily fish, nuts, seeds, avocado, olive oil.

If you're a nutritional therapist, you may favour a specific dietary approach, such as the keto diet or intermittent fasting, but personally I keep things as simple and uncomplicated as possible, at least initially. Here are a few manageable, easily assembled meals I often suggest:

Breakfast

- Full-fat plain yogurt (cows/goats/coconut) with a large spoonful of almond butter, seeds and berries.
- Porridge made with plant-based milk and a little cacao powder, nuts/nut butter, seeds, berries.

Lunch

- Omelette with spinach, tomatoes, mushrooms and a salad or with peas, spring onion and feta cheese and a salad.
- Leftovers from the night before.
- Falafel and hummus or, alternatively, a tin of tuna, with avocado, cherry tomatoes, beetroot and salad leaves.

Evening meal

- Salmon, chicken or tofu, broccoli and red pepper with garlic, lemon and tamari with brown rice (from a ready-cooked pouch for convenience).
- Bean and veggie chilli (make double for a second meal) with brown rice or quinoa and guacamole.
- Chicken or halloumi in lime and chilli with oven-roasted peppers, aubergine, sweet potatoes and a green salad.

If they feel in need of a sweet treat after a meal then dark chocolate will provide some magnesium and antioxidants and maybe also help stimulate some feel-good endorphins.

As grief sometimes comes in waves, you could suggest to your client that when they are having a better day, they batch-cook so that they then have a few healthy meals in the freezer to use when the grief hits again and they feel less up to cooking. This may avert resorting to takeaways on a bad day.

Other considerations

It may be useful to point out to your client that many people experiencing anxiety during the grieving process can have a heightened sensitivity to caffeine, increasing HPA axis activity (see above). Alcohol, too, and recreational drugs, which your grieving client may turn to in order to help them cope with their emotional discomfort, will potentially interfere with neurotransmitter balance in the brain, disrupting blood sugar balance and depleting the very nutrients important for a healthy stress response.

NUTRIENTS THAT ARE HELPFUL FOR STRESS AND ANXIETY DURING GRIEF
Magnesium

Magnesium is a key mineral for the stress of grief. Magnesium-rich foods include nuts, seeds, salmon, mackerel, tofu, leafy greens, beans, quinoa and dark chocolate. In addition, it can be very helpful to supplement magnesium, especially as many clients will probably not be getting enough from their diet. I usually supplement magnesium either as part of a complex for nervous system support or in the form of glycinate, which is especially appropriate if a grieving client is suffering with insomnia, anxiety, PTSD or adrenal fatigue.

Stress rapidly consumes magnesium, which is unfortunate as the body really needs magnesium if it's to respond effectively to stress.

Studies have highlighted the relationship between serum cortisol and magnesium, showing that the higher the magnesium, the lower the cortisol.[3] Depending on the client, it may also be necessary for you to bear in mind that many medications deplete magnesium, as does the intake of alcohol, caffeine and soft drinks.

In his article 'Magnesium: The missing link in mental health?' James Greenblatt reports that some of the highest levels of magnesium in the body are found in the central nervous system and that magnesium is crucial for a balanced brain: 'It's known, for example, that magnesium interacts with GABA receptors, supporting the calming actions of this neurotransmitter. Magnesium also keeps glutamate – an excitatory neurotransmitter – within healthy limits.' Magnesium is also crucial for the role it plays in the pituitary gland, regulating the release of the hormone ACTH, which then stimulates the release of cortisol in the adrenal glands. Magnesium then helps to maintain a healthy response to ACTH in the adrenal glands, keeping cortisol release within a normal range. To further highlight the importance of magnesium, those with higher levels were also found to have good levels of serotonin in the cerebrospinal fluid, according to Greenblatt.[4] And in a recent meta-analysis of 11 studies on magnesium and depression, people with the lowest intake of magnesium were 81 per cent more likely to be depressed than those with the highest intake.[5]

B vitamins

B vitamins (found in foods such as brown rice, poultry, eggs, dairy produce, legumes, seeds and nuts, and dark, leafy vegetables) can play a beneficial role in reducing anxiety and improving mood, and are therefore definitely worth consideration for your grieving client. One study found there was evidence that B group vitamin

---

3   Dmitrašinović *et al.*, 2016; Savonix, 2018; Schutten *et al.*, 2021
4   Greenblatt, 2016
5   Li *et al.*, 2016

supplementation (either alone or with a multi vitamin) may benefit those with depression, anxiety and stress.[6] It is also thought that B12 is especially important for anxiety, depression and problems with focus, memory and energy – all of which can occur during grief. Most good-quality multis have methylated B vitamins, so this is how I tend to supplement them in most cases when working with a grieving client.

Methylated nutrients carry and transfer methyl groups from one compound to another. This process, called methylation, is necessary for the proper functioning of the body and overall health. Signs of poor methylation include anxiety, depression and insomnia, which also occur during the grieving process and which we are attempting to support. If you use a supplement with unmethylated B vitamins, it takes a few more enzyme steps before the methyl groups are available. However, this slower delivery may be beneficial to people who are sensitive to methylated nutrients.

Vitamin C

Vitamin C is going to be helpful for any inflammation caused by the stress of grief. It is also important for the nervous system and the adrenals, helping the body to better manage cortisol levels. One study on the role of vitamin C stated that 'vitamin C deficiency is widely associated with stress-related diseases' and that taking a vitamin C supplement may improve mood and reduce anxiety.[7] Vitamin C is also supportive of the heart and the immune system, and we know that grief can affect immunity and that some traumatic losses can lead to a predisposition towards cancer and heart issues. Therefore, recommending foods rich in vitamin C, along with supplementation, is definitely worth considering for some grieving clients.

---

6   Young *et al.*, 2019
7   Moritz *et al.*, 2020

Vitamin D

It's well known that a large percentage of the population are deficient in vitamin D, especially during the winter, and that there is a correlation between low vitamin D levels and higher rates of anxiety, low mood and poor immunity. I'm sure many of us suggest supplementation to the majority of our clients, and this is going to be particularly relevant to one who is grieving.

Omega 3

There are numerous studies that show omega 3 supports brain function, so it makes sense to encourage your client to eat oily fish or to take a supplement. This may potentially be helpful not only for any anxiety and depression during grief but also for any issues with brain fog and memory that have come to the fore during the grieving process. It's also important for heart health – as highlighted in Chapter 3, grief can take its toll on the heart.

Botanicals

Botanicals such as passionflower, valerian, lemon balm, camomile, lavender and hops are definitely worth considering, especially where anxiety or PTSD is present. Their ability to calm the nervous system and aid sleep makes them particularly useful during grief. Many supplement companies provide a combination of these ingredients in a complex, and so it's a good idea to look at these. As is so often the case, what works well for one client may not work so well for another, so there may be some trial and error involved.

Adaptogens

Adaptogens are herbs, often used as part of the ayurvedic tradition, that have been used for thousands of years to balance hormones, alleviate stress and fight fatigue. Adaptogens respond to what the body needs: they can calm you down and boost your energy at the same time without overstimulating – in other words, adaptogens adapt. The adaptogen that is perhaps most appropriate during grief is ashwagandha as it has proven anti-stress properties. It works by supporting the adrenal system to mediate the body's response to stress. In one study, participants who took ashwagandha for 60 days lowered their cortisol levels by almost 30 per cent.[8] Ashwagandha can be used on its own or as part of a complex designed to support the stress and anxiety that may be experienced during grief.

What to use for depression

As antidepressants are so frequently prescribed to the bereaved, it's quite important, in my view, that we have a viable alternative to offer, and one that has undergone scientific trials. Many of our clients will welcome an effective alternative, especially if it doesn't have side effects, begins to work quickly, can be stopped without any withdrawal symptoms and won't make them feel like a zombie.

Obviously, a good diet, optimal vitamin D and omega 3 can all help, but we have to acknowledge that not all depression can be remedied through just treating the physical – it is inevitable that if you've lost someone you love dearly, you will naturally feel depressed to a greater or lesser degree – so there are limits to what we (and doctors) can do. However, there is one particular supplement I have used for years with clients who suffer with mild to moderate depression, and I now use it with grieving clients who would like a natural alternative to antidepressants.

Crocus sativus

Saffron, a spice derived from the flower of *Crocus sativus*, has now undergone several trials examining its antidepressant effects and, in a recent meta-analysis, was confirmed to be effective for the treatment of major depression. The results revealed that:

---

8   Chandrasekhar, Kapoor and Anishetty, 2012

In the systematic review, six studies were identified. In the placebo-comparison trials, saffron had large treatment effects and, when compared with antidepressant medications, had similar anti-depressant efficacy. Saffron's antidepressant effects potentially are due to its serotonergic, antioxidant, anti-inflammatory, neuro-endocrine and neuroprotective effects.[9]

There are many similar studies to be found that support the efficacy of *Crocus sativus*. I use this as my go-to supplement for clients with depression, whether grief-related or otherwise. Unlike conventional antidepressants, it starts to take effect quickly (within a day or so in my experience), doesn't cause grogginess and can be stopped without any withdrawal symptoms. However, to reiterate, it's important to manage your client's expectations. Depression in grief is caused by the pain of a loved one's absence, and no antidepressant – natural or otherwise – can change that.

There are other options, such as 5HPT – I sometimes combine this with *Crocus sativus* – and St John's Wort, although this has the disadvantage of taking several weeks before it begins to be effective.

Note: Always check for contraindications.

Insomnia

This is often such a big issue in grief. Grief and trauma are hard enough to deal with, but if you can't sleep and you're exhausted as a result, everything just feels even worse, sometimes to the point of deep despair. Working on calming the nervous system will undoubtedly help. Magnesium is of paramount importance in helping with sleep – especially in the form of glycinate. Worth consideration too are the botanicals mentioned above and also GABA and L-theanine. A study titled 'GABA and L-theanine mixture decreases sleep latency and improves NREM sleep' concluded: 'GABA/l-theanine mixture has a positive synergistic effect on sleep quality and duration as compared

---

9   Lopresti and Drummond, 2014, p.517

to the GABA or l-theanine alone.'[10] There are plenty of complexes available to support better sleep, so it's a question of finding the best one for your client's individual needs. Breathing techniques, as already indicated, can also be helpful for sleep, as can sleep apps.

A role for nutritional medicine in PTSD

Ben Brown wrote an interesting article entitled 'PTSD: Building resilience to trauma-induced mental health issues with a functional medicine approach' in the July 2020 edition of *IHCAN* (Integrative Healthcare and Applied Nutrition) magazine. He believes there is a huge opportunity for integrative care to reduce the suffering involved in PTSD.[11]

He says:

> Dietary change and personal nutrient-based supplements would seem to be a logical approach to the management of PTSD, considering their ability to improve several aspects of mental and physical health relevant to the disorder, such as mood, depressive symptoms and cardiometabolic disease. However current evidence is limited to mostly observational studies. PTSD symptom severity has been associated with a less nutritious diet and emotional eating disorders.

Brown cites a case report published by the Maryland University of Integrated Health which included personalized supplementation (amino acids, a multi vitamin, zinc, vitamin C, gamma-linolenic acid and magnesium) and a low-GI diet. This resulted in marked clinical improvement in a patient with PTSD who was responding poorly to medication. Despite a lack of research on such personalized nutritional treatments, there is evidence for individual interventions as follows.

---

10   Kim *et al.*, 2019, p.65
11   Brown, 2020

Broad spectrum micronutrients

There is striking evidence, according to Brown's article, to show that broad spectrum micronutrients may significantly prevent the development of psychiatric symptoms after trauma. Overall, he says, broad spectrum micronutrient therapy appears to be a safe, cost-effective intervention that could have an effect on reducing risk for the development of PTSD as well as mitigating symptoms post-trauma (the latter being potentially relevant to a grieving client diagnosed with PTSD).

Vitamin D

Deficiency may increase vulnerability to PTSD, especially in certain genotypes. We know how prevalent vitamin D deficiency is in the general population and how it can be helpful for mental health generally (see earlier in this chapter).

Omega 3 fatty acids

Brown states that not only are low blood levels of omega 3 associated with increased risk of PTSD, supplementation for 12 weeks was shown to significantly reduce PTSD symptoms in accident-injured patients admitted to intensive care. Although we are looking specifically at PTSD in grief, this does suggest omega 3 supplementation could help, especially as it is known to reduce inflammatory markers.

Note: While I think it is worth considering all of the above, it won't be the case that every grieving client with PTSD has the above deficiencies; I didn't, either before or after trauma.

N-acetylcysteine (NAC)

Brown says NAC has been shown to be a useful treatment for PTSD, including depressive symptoms.

Cannabidiol (CBD)

As CBD has been shown to be involved in the regulation of mood, it may also be a potential target for PTSD, as it has been associated with reduced anxiety and sleep symptoms.

Chronic health issues that may have grief as an underlying cause

While the focus in this chapter has mainly been on the most pressing symptoms you are likely to see in your grieving clients, it is wise to always have in mind the revelations in Chapter 3 regarding the implications for serious health outcomes, such as cancer and heart disease. These conditions may not necessarily present themselves in the early months of grief, or even the early years, but they could develop insidiously over time. The trauma of certain losses can change the body at a cellular level that the client won't be aware of.

Although there is no evidence (as yet) for whether the stress of grief impacts Covid-19 outcomes, there is evidence that stress affects immune function and raises inflammatory levels. My strong belief, based on personal experience with regard to my husband – a bereaved father who died of Covid yet had no known underlying health conditions – is that it potentially can do so, when the grief is traumatic. And the lungs, which as we know are the organs most affected by Covid, are associated with grief according to Traditional Chinese Medicine.

Supporting immune function and a more targeted approach to lowering inflammation with specific supplements is definitely worthy of consideration. You may also want to focus on heart health if you have any indications that this might be appropriate. And gently informing your client about some of the ways grief can potentially affect their long-term physical health, without frightening them, might mean that they have an incentive to keep looking after themselves beyond the time they work with you.

Being in possession of all the research outlined gives us a good reason to ensure that we not only always recommend an anti-inflammatory diet, but we work tirelessly to bring the stress of grief under control, so that we do our utmost to lower the chances of our client going on to develop a very serious and possibly life-limiting health issue. However, while it's important to do all we can, please always bear in mind that some outcomes are beyond our control despite our best efforts and remain complex for reasons beyond our understanding.

CHAPTER 10

Recommendations for Your Grieving Client

In Chapter 9, we focused specifically on nutritional medicine; in this chapter, we will look at some grief coaching tools that any practitioner could use or suggest either in or outside their sessions. The ideas in this chapter will be varied and based on those I personally used to support myself through grief, as well as recommendations I've subsequently seen to have worked well for my clients. Some ideas work for certain people better than others, and although we can use our discernment when we suggest an idea based on our assessment of a client's needs, if you suggest something and the client doesn't find it helpful, then swiftly move on to something else. There is more of an immediacy when working with grief – we want to offer some respite as soon as possible. Using my holistic grief wheel gives me an immediate idea of the areas of grief most in need of attention.

THE HOLISTIC GRIEF WHEEL

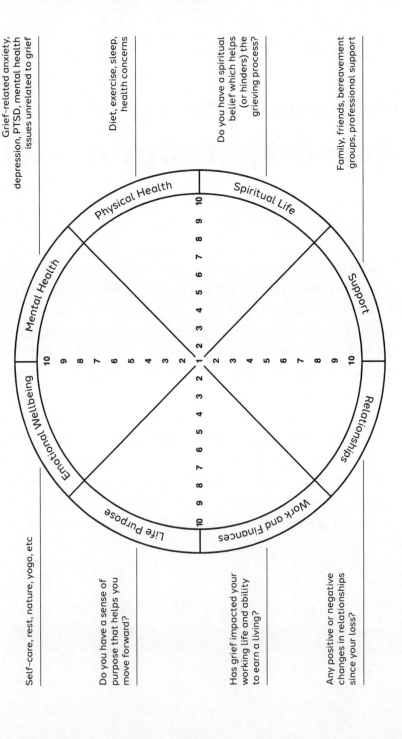

Grief-related anxiety, depression, PTSD, mental health issues unrelated to grief

Diet, exercise, sleep, health concerns

Do you have a spiritual belief which helps (or hinders) the grieving process?

Family, friends, bereavement groups, professional support

Self-care, rest, nature, yoga, etc

Do you have a sense of purpose that helps you move forward?

Has grief impacted your working life and ability to earn a living?

Any positive or negative changes in relationships since your loss?

Physical Health

Spiritual Life

Mental Health

Support

Emotional Wellbeing

Relationships

Life Purpose

Work and Finances

As a wellbeing coach, I usually ask a client to fill out a coaching wheel before we begin sessions as it provides an opportunity to open up a conversation and to then promptly home in on specific areas. For those of you who are not familiar with a coaching wheel, it encourages self-enquiry in a client and gives an overview of how satisfied they are with their life and in what areas they might want to set and prioritize some goals. It would obviously not be appropriate to use a wheel in this form for a grieving client. However, inspired by a suggestion from a friend who I trained in wellbeing coaching with, I have now created a wheel specifically to use with grieving clients. I have chosen eight segments that I feel impact grief the most and invite a client to give each a score – 10 being the best it could be and 1 being the worst it could be. They then draw a line across each segment, creating a wheel.

Ideally, with a normal coaching wheel, after several (or many) sessions, you aim to end up with every section being given high scores so that the wheel is less wonky than it perhaps was initially. This will probably be less achievable with a grieving client, and you may find some very low scoring, in which case reassure them that this is to be expected, but re-scoring the wheel after several sessions may actually reveal surprising improvements in certain areas, and this can be used to encourage them to hope that they could also make similar progress in another area. That said, some areas won't show any change and may even score lower on a second or third scoring. Reassurance that this is normal but that there is still every hope that any area can improve is key.

Once you have their wheel and you're in a session with them, it can be a good idea to begin by asking about the higher-scoring segments first. In Jodie's wheel in Chapter 6, she scored herself very highly in both 'spiritual life' and 'life purpose', so this was a good place to start a conversation and quickly gave me some insights about her. By contrast, other sections did not score nearly so well, especially 'mental health' and 'emotional wellbeing', so immediately these were flagged up to me, which I found helpful for providing me with an awareness of where we might need to focus.

Sometimes, at the end of a session I will ask a client if they'd like to choose a section of the wheel to look at next time. Interestingly, it's not always one I might expect them to choose. The idea isn't necessarily to look at every single section, though it's quite possible you will touch on all of them, intentionally or not. And, of course, you don't have to continue using the wheel if you feel the sessions are flowing organically. It is, after all, just an optional tool to serve you and your client.

So, when would you give the wheel to your grieving client? This will depend. If you know about their loss, you could send it through before their first session, along with your 'terms of engagement' form. If you do this, a little explanation will be necessary, along the lines of: 'This is just to give us a starting point for where we might most want to focus to best support you through your loss. There is no right or wrong to this and it's to be expected that some scores won't be very high at this stage.' Also, don't forget to explain how to score it. You want to do everything to encourage their understanding that this is designed to help you to help them, as well as highlighting for themselves any area that particularly needs to be addressed. At all costs, you want to avoid this being a stressful task that adds to any anxiety, although this will be unlikely as long as you explain its purpose clearly. Alternatively, you can fill it in together during a session if you have a client who is especially suffering with brain fog or feeling overwhelmed. If you don't know in advance that someone is bereaved, or you feel it's too much information to send through in addition to your usual paperwork, then just suggest during a session that you would like to email it through so that you can look at it together next time.

To sum up, this can be a very useful tool for initiating a conversation around a sensitive subject, which you may feel unsure about how to broach. It can effectively highlight any shifts that may occur over the course of your sessions, which could be encouraging for your client to see in a visual form. It also helps you to identify quickly and graphically the areas of grief that most need attention.

If you'd like a copy of the holistic grief wheel, please contact me via my website: www.vanessamay.co.uk.

A TOOL TO MONITOR GRIEF INTENSITY AND THE ABILITY TO COPE

Joanne Cacciatore, who wrote *Bearing the Unbearable: Love, Loss, and the Heartbreaking Path of Grief*, says that when she works with a bereaved person, she has no agenda, no goals, no clinical objectives or treatment plan. She has no particular destination in mind; she is just with them as they move through grief. Her only aim is to 'help them feel the complete, unedited version of their particular story'.[1] She uses the following tool for assessment:

Grief intensity (1 least, 10 most)

1	2	3	4	5	6	7	8	9	10

Ability to cope with grief (1 least, 10 most)

1	2	3	4	5	6	7	8	9	10

This approach of just simply being with someone in their grief has, I believe, great merit. Most of us as wellness practitioners do tend, however, to work in a more goal-focused way – that is, giving some-one strategies or treatments to make some measurable difference to their suffering. If we are able to find room for both approaches – being and doing – then I feel that strikes a good balance, and it's certainly how I try to work. The above tool can be a useful one to gauge just how intense your client's grief really is – it's clear and concise, and you may find unanticipated scores with clients who are

---

1   Cacciatore, 2017, p.59

adept at putting on a socially acceptable face. They could be swans furiously paddling to stay afloat underneath the water...

OTHER TOOLS YOU CAN SUGGEST TO YOUR GRIEVING CLIENT

There are many suggestions I offer my clients, some of which I will share here. A few may seem obvious to you, but perhaps not to a grieving client who is struggling to make sense of their new situation. I find it can sometimes be helpful to ask them to fill their own personal 'healing' or 'self-care' basket – choose whatever term you feel might resonate best with them. It can be good to encourage them to write down (or draw) what's in their 'basket' to share with you next time. You can start this off by asking what helps ease their suffering. They may say that nothing does, but then you find out they feel better for being out in nature, eating a nutritious breakfast or taking a magnesium bath – these would then go into their 'self-care basket'. The idea is to get them to keep adding to the list so that, while we're not downplaying how difficult their circumstances might be, we help them to see that there are things that can help lessen their suffering. Our aim is to help them find ways to soothe the soul, nurture their wellbeing and find some purpose and meaning in life – in spite of what has happened to them.

Journaling

I suggest this a lot. Writing can be an excellent way to process what has happened, and there are plenty of studies that show it's beneficial for anxiety, depression and heart health. Apparently, 10–15 minutes of creative writing reduces cortisol.[2] It's vital to point out to your client that no one needs to read what they write, so that they feel free to get anything they want to out of their system and down on paper.

---

2   Baikie and Wilhelm, 2005; Harris, 2014

Writing without a filter is key so as not to be hindered by what people might think. This then averts any feeling of exposure, inhibition or unnecessary vulnerability, which could be triggering for them. They can always shred or burn what they've written afterwards if they're worried someone might come across it – and indeed this in itself can feel like a healing act of letting go of any unnecessary burdens. Journaling can, of course, be done on a laptop or phone and then deleted, but there is something about the tangible act of writing on paper that seems to make this a more powerful exercise.

Writing for many grieving clients can be a great form of pain relief and a way to metabolize their experience. It was definitely the best form of grief therapy for me, which then took the form of my book *Love Untethered*. Most people won't write a book, but some may do, or they may choose to write a blog on their experience. Although being 'seen' in this way isn't for everyone, you can be a great cheerleader for your client if you observe that their writing is providing a little light in the dark for them. I have had a few clients who have asked if they can share their writing with me, and I have felt incredibly honoured when this has happened.

Writing can be a potentially helpful tool for trauma as it's said that writing about your trauma can give you back your voice, enabling you to express what you may have been unable to articulate at the time due to the shock you were experiencing. Witnessing your own story by getting everything you're feeling down on paper can create a safe distance from what happened, and that can be a positive step forward. Stepping away by taking regular breaks is recommended, and if it feels triggering, then havening can really help to keep them in the present (see Chapter 4). If, however, you can see writing is having an unforeseen detrimental effect on your client at that particular stage of their grief, then do not encourage them to continue in the hope that this may be overcome. Writing about pain is not for everyone. It will help some but not others.

If your client doesn't seem to find that writing in the ways outlined above is for them, but you still think that getting their feelings down on the page could help them, then another suggestion that I often make is to write a letter to the person who has died, telling them anything they feel they need to say but perhaps didn't, for whatever reason. Most people find this exercise incredibly cathartic. Another idea, if you think they might be open to it, is to follow this by writing back to themselves, as their loved one. I did this as part of a Helping Parents Heal group of bereaved parents, and it was incredible how the words from our children just flowed from the pen and felt immensely comforting, enhancing our connection with them and our continuing bond. Writing isn't for everyone but, in my experience, even some of the clients who are initially reluctant to give it a go can often find some benefit. Never push it, though; if they're not keen, move on to something else.

Breathwork and meditation

We've already discussed how breathing techniques can be really helpful for calming the nervous system and for sleep, too. Some of you may be able to incorporate breathwork into your sessions. You can also suggest meditation to your client. Meditation is now considered mainstream as a way of helping with the stress of our modern-day lives, so it makes sense that this could be extended to the stress of grief, too. It is generally accepted that meditation may reduce anxiety, boost the immune system and increase concentration and focus. It's also good for living in the present moment, which can give someone who is grieving a break from endlessly ruminating on what happened in the past or fixated on feelings of hopelessness when they consider the future. It is even thought to provide the nervous system with a rest that is five times deeper than sleep,[3] so it's worth suggesting if insomnia is an issue. Meditation can also help with managing other physical symptoms of grief, such as muscle tension and headaches.

---

3   Hyman, 2019

Using the breath will help soothe the nervous system and promote a better sense of wellbeing.

There are plenty of meditations available on YouTube and you could also suggest the Calm[4] and Headspace[5] apps. I found it helpful to use guided meditations and visualizations during early grief. Focusing on specific instructions is sometimes easier at such a challenging time, when your mind understandably wanders to upsetting thoughts or images. I found a ten-minute chakra meditation was just the right length for me,[6] but you may have your own suggestions.

Please note, however, that although, as someone with PTSD, I didn't find breathing techniques or meditation problematic, there are some people that might. In certain cases, they can trigger flashbacks or dissociation. Also, any meditation – either on an app, YouTube or with a practitioner – that focuses on going to a 'happy place' may jar with many clients, so recommend appropriately.

Essential oils

If you work with essential oils as an aromatherapist, then you won't need convincing that essential oils can provide a lovely way to support emotional and energetic wellbeing during grief. The smell from certain essential oils directly impacts the limbic system, the region of the brain that activates our fight-or-flight response, potentially helping with the release of emotional trauma. As we know, when people have been traumatized, this is the part of the brain that is the most affected. Essential oils affect the hypothalamus and pituitary gland, which, once stimulated, release hormones into the body. For example, lavender essential oil can have a positive effect on sleep, by relaxing the muscles and allowing you to fall asleep more easily; this

---

4   www.calm.com
5   www.headspace.com
6   Heslop, 2019

is a decision made by the body in the limbic system once the lavender essential oil vapour has been inhaled.[7]

Lavender and rose can be used for anxiety and restful sleep, and rose geranium and orange are uplifting oils and so provide a little boost. The oils I most use are two doTERRA blends.[8] One is called Peace: Reassuring blend, which can be helpful for anxiety, and the other is called Console: Comforting blend, which is indicated for grief. I sometimes put them in a diffuser, but, more often than not, I rub them together in the palm of my hands and inhale. When I do this, I feel a noticeable difference and a subtle shift in how I'm feeling. There are safety issues with some essential oils so, if necessary, remind your client to seek advice from a qualified aromatherapist.

For some of your grieving clients, the use of oils may be a suggestion that appeals and can be part of their healing basket of tools, whether to use at home or as part of a relaxing massage with an aromatherapist.

Sound healing

There has been an increased interest in sound healing recently, and if you have a client who you feel might like this, then it could be a very nice healing tool for them to use during the grieving process. Sound healing is an ancient meditative practice that originated in Tibet 2000 years ago, where you bathe in sound waves. Different musical implements may be used to create healing vibrations around the body in a meditative state. Singing bowl therapists use quartz crystal bowls and gongs tuned at strategic frequencies for healing different parts of the body and mind, potentially helping with anxiety and depression. Although there are actual places you can go for a sound bath, you can listen to crystal 'singing' bowls on YouTube (I like the 11-minute Chakra Tune Up from Temple Sounds[9]). There is a

---

7   Scentered, 2020
8   www.doterra.com/GB/en_GB
9   www.youtube.com/watch?v=-ar9vsmFhJU

different bowl, and therefore sound, for each chakra, and so you can visualize the colour for each one and may even feel something physically in each area of the body where the chakra is centred. Sound baths have the potential to provide a grieving client with a 'reset' at times when they're feeling overwhelmed.

Solfeggio frequencies are tones of sound that are purported to promote the health of the mind, body and spirit. The frequencies balance and aid healing by the effect the sounds have on the conscious and unconscious mind. Physician and researcher Dr Joseph Puleo rediscovered Solfeggio frequencies in the 1970s, bringing their benefits back into public awareness.[10] In his research, he used mathematical numeral reduction to identify six measurable tones that bring the body back into balance and aid in healing. Our cells appear to be responsive to frequency and vibration, so the potential for these frequencies to be used as a component in healing grief or trauma is worth considering. At the very least, they are very relaxing to listen to. There are plenty of Solfeggio frequencies to be found on YouTube.

Nature

I included nature in Chapter 3, but it's worth mentioning again here because its benefits cannot be underestimated for someone who is grieving. Walking in nature is known to help with our mental wellbeing, but even if your client just sits on a bench in the park or in their own garden, that will also provide benefits, especially if they ground themselves by placing their bare feet on the earth and look up at the sky.

Gardening is another suggestion you could make. Getting your hands in the soil, helping things to grow, tending to them and watching them bloom is definitely therapeutic. I have a grief coaching client who would say her garden has played a key role in surviving her loss.

---

10 BetterSleep, n.d.

Grief yoga

The benefits of yoga during grief have already discussed in Chapter 3. I recommend this to nearly all my clients, specifically Yoga with Adriene, who has Yoga for Grief, Yoga for PTSD and Yoga for Anxiety.[11] These don't involve complex poses but are mainly focused on breathing and gentle stretching, and are only around an achievable 25 minutes. Of course, you can suggest a local class if you know of one, but it's sometimes so much easier in early grief to just switch on your laptop and not have to interact with other people.

Creativity

Creativity can be a great outlet during grief. Pain needs expression, and creativity can provide a place for it to go so that it doesn't end up residing in the body, wreaking potential havoc. Letting the pain live in writing, art, music and other creative outlets means the pain is channelled somewhere, and this can aid healing. You could ask your client if some of the following spark any kind of interest: painting, photography, knitting, mosaics or pottery. These are all activities where you can lose yourself for a few hours and claim a little respite from grief, with the added bonus of feeling a sense of accomplishment for what you produce.

Singing also provides many benefits, including lowering stress levels and aiding sleep, so joining a choir might be another suggestion you could make.

Dance/movement can have therapeutic potential, too – not focusing on technique or performance but instead on the creative, expressive process. Dance and movement encourage a sense of flow and very much bring us out of our heads and into our bodies, helping to ground us and to develop breath support.

A creative activity centred around the person who has passed away is something I frequently suggest. Some like to sort through

---

11   https://yogawithadriene.com

photographs and give a framed collection to others who loved them. I found making framed collages very therapeutic. I used photos of my son, flowers I had pressed from the funeral bouquet and sentences printed off from poems that resonated with me. This is an idea I now pass on.

Vision boards are also a good creative activity. A vision board is a collection of images that, in the case of someone who is grieving, might provide a little comfort and hope. When first bereaved, my existing vision board no longer made any sense to me, so, given time, I created a different one with photographs, poems and affirmations. The latter were gentle and realistic but also hopeful. As our feelings during the grieving process change, it's possible a poem, photo or affirmation which resonated at one point may not at another. Therefore, it's a good idea to regularly change what's on the vision board to reflect current feelings. For some clients, especially the visual ones, a vision board may be a positive and creative project that could give them some enjoyment, as well as a little hope, at a very difficult time.

Continuing bonds

The continuing bonds theory was discussed in Chapter 5, but to briefly recap, remaining connected to a loved one facilitates the ability of the bereaved to cope with loss and the subsequent changes to their lives. Healthy grieving is no longer believed to be resolved by detaching from the person who has died and 'finding closure', but instead by creating a new relationship with them. The relationship is never over, simply changed. This can be an important part of coming to terms with their physical absence and one that doesn't necessarily need to include a spiritual belief.

It's natural for a bereaved person to wonder with every passing year how their loved one might have looked, what they would now be doing or how they would have changed. This can be painful, but that pain can be eased somewhat if they are able to share those thoughts with someone. Being able to talk about how the person they have lost would have enjoyed a new film, loved a new place, or what they would have made of the pandemic (if they died before it began) can be an important part of the healing process and coming to terms with the fact that they will never be able to interact with them in physical form again. It's a way of keeping the person who has died always with them – and for many this can soften the pain. It's making the decision that the relationship doesn't have to be frozen in time or locked in the past. If there isn't a spiritual belief, then the relationship can continue by carrying the love they have for them in their heart and by honouring in some of the ways outlined below.

However, if your grieving client has a spiritual belief that the soul lives on after physical death (and never underestimate just how many people do), then they will be open, in addition, to continuing their relationship through 'conversations', by being open to signs from their loved ones or possibly through consulting a medium. The connection between the bereaved living soul and the soul who is no longer in physical form can evolve to another level, and this, in some cases, can prove a key way of surviving loss for the one still living. Just as people and relationships grow and evolve in life, so too can they keep growing and evolving after death. If someone has this belief, they will 'feel' their loved one and know they are close by. Whatever you personally believe, it's key to respect whatever may be true for your client. Don't underestimate how this could be what's allowing them to take tentative steps towards a future that is without the physical presence of their loved one but which could be sustained by a spiritual bond of boundless love.

I always discuss the continuing bonds theory with a grieving client – with or without the spiritual element – and use it as a starting point to discuss ways they might like to honour the person they have lost.

There are some that bring a light so great to the world that even after they have gone, the light remains.

UNKNOWN

Suggestions for honouring the person who has died

Finding ways – both big and small – that the person who is grieving can honour who they have lost helps with acceptance of the physical loss by continuing the bond and finding a tangible expression for their love. There are many ways to do this, and here are a few ideas that 1, and others, have found helpful and which you could discuss with your grieving client:

- A memorial bench – either in a local park, beauty spot or, if allowed, at the place of burial.
- A slate plaque with an inscription. This could be for the garden or possibly a more public space.
- Planting a rose bush or a tree.
- A memory book where everyone who knew the person can write a message.
- Making collages (see 'Creativity' above).
- Candles – whether lighting them in the home beside a photo or lighting one in a church or other place of worship.
- Collections that may or not be directly connected to the loved ones. For example, anything with the initial of their name, feathers you find, heart-shaped pebbles, crystal angels, etc.
- Wear their clothes or jewellery. To someone who hasn't experienced deep grief, this may sound odd, but it can feel incredibly comforting to a bereaved person and it's natural in early grief to smell their clothes as a way of trying to keep the connection to their physical being.
- Writing a letter (see 'Journaling' above) or a poem, or writing the story of their life.
- A small table or an area of the home dedicated to the loved one where there are photos, candles and any objects associated with the person or collected by the griever. Again, this may sound morbid if you haven't had a life-shattering

loss, but if someone has, then this can continue the bond and bring a much-needed sense of peace and comfort.

- Continue with something they enjoyed. Support their favourite football team, take up photography, watch their favourite film or TV series – anything that keeps the connection in a healing way.

- Many bereaved people seem to find it helps them to give back in some way and may choose to raise money for a charity associated with the person they have lost. This can be done by a fundraising event or by setting up a tribute page on a website such as Much Loved,[12] where donations to the chosen charity can be made, as well as providing a place where friends and family can write a tribute.

- Dedicate a star to the person who has died. Although you could argue that you can't really buy a star, many feel that it's a lovely idea to associate a star with someone they loved, and it's also something that can be shared among friends and family who can then search for it in the night sky.

- Set up a website dedicated to the person who has died, where everyone who wants to can post photos and stories.

- Put together an e-book using Canva,[13] asking friends and family to contribute memories, stories and photos. This is a great 'project' to do in the dreaded days leading up to a birthday, anniversary or Christmas or other festival. It can be uplifting to hear stories that they haven't heard before. This tribute can then be shared, uniting those that loved the person, keeping the bond alive.

- At Christmas time or at another festival, fill a trolley with the favourite food of the loved one and donate it to a homeless organization.

- Keep something as a reminder of them in a prominent

---

12 www.muchloved.com
13 www.canva.com

spot. It may be something as simple as leaving their shoes or coat in the hall, or their watch by the bed. I keep a jar of Marmite (which has our son's name on – a present in his Christmas stocking one year) permanently on the kitchen table, like a place setting. That way he is always with us when we sit down for a meal, acting as evidence that he lived here, was part of our family and always will be.

Post-traumatic growth

Following on from the healing power of continuing bonds, cultivating post-traumatic growth after a loss may, in some cases, be possible. (David Kessler discusses this in his book *Finding Meaning*.[14]) This mainly applies to a profound life-changing loss, as such intense pain can shift a bereaved person's perception of life on a very deep level, and while it's important not to assume this will happen with your client, it is possible to grow after a tragedy. In fact, from my personal perspective, it's possible to experience the continued pain of ongoing grief and PTSD, while at the same time experiencing post-traumatic growth – one does not appear to necessarily preclude the other. Post-traumatic growth can include discovering a new purpose in life, helping others who have experienced a similar tragedy, becoming more compassionate, a deepening spirituality, discovering an inner strength you perhaps didn't know you had, and developing stronger relationships.

Do, however, watch out for a client who seems overly determined to turn their pain into purpose and possesses a driven desire to transform it into something meaningful. It's not healthy to do this if it bypasses the healing of their grief and trauma, and you may need to reassure them that sometimes it's necessary to just sit with the pain, excruciating as that might be, and that it isn't something that's

---

14 Kessler, 2019

'negative' and needs avoiding. It is, in fact, an essential part of their ongoing healing.

'Healthy grieving' entails moving towards eventually integrating the loss into our lives; it's about finding meaning and purpose but not doing so by avoiding the discomfort of grief, as that will only prolong the pain. Healthy grief is ideally about finding the balance between grieving fully while living fully. You may come across some clients who want to avoid difficult feelings at all costs, but if the challenging feelings of grief are avoided, then they're likely to resurface at a later date, potentially affecting various aspects of health. As we know, the body keeps the score. If you have a client with the tendency to avoid discomfort, you can perhaps explain that only by moving through the pain will it be possible to release it. That said, in some cases where there has been significant trauma, feelings may get suppressed because they feel too 'unsafe' to be felt, in which case the client may benefit from specialist trauma therapies, as previously discussed.

While first and foremost, I encourage compassionately witnessing someone's grief and holding space for the client without trying to fix them, if and when the time is right, you can gently introduce the idea of post-traumatic growth and explain how finding meaning after a loss may be helpful to their healing. Finding meaning in life post-loss doesn't completely take away the pain but it can perhaps be likened to adding a cushion. It's useful to bear in mind that post-traumatic growth is not the same as personal development. In 'normal' life, personal development is to be aspired to for many aspects of growth, but when grief and trauma are present, matters may be far more complex and a balance needs to be sought. If your client is not at the stage of being ready to consider the possibility of post-traumatic growth, you can encourage them, as follows, to seek some comfort in small pleasures.

Small pleasures

Once your client is a little way into their grief journey, you may want to gently encourage a hope that some aspects of life can still be enjoyed – not in any way to minimize what has happened to them or to encourage any unrealistic plans and goals, but just by gently getting them to focus on small pleasures. That might simply be sitting outside on a sunny day with a friend, a slice of their favourite cake or watching a good series on Netflix. We tend to mark our lives by the big tangible milestones, such as graduations, weddings or career changes. In grief, these milestones may either no longer be possible or may have lost their appeal or relevance, now seeming unimportant in comparison with the loss of an important person. So, when things feel uncertain for your client, it can be reassuring and more achievable to focus on small things in their life that may bring a little comfort and pleasure.

Observing nature by planting some bulbs in a pot and waiting for the flowers to grow is often a suggestion I make. Getting outside for a walk is something I constantly advocate. To literally put one foot in front of the other, to take one step at a time, symbolizes the emotional effort it sometimes takes to get through each day when someone is on an often unforgiving journey of grief and can provide not insignificant benefits to a fragile sense of wellbeing. As mentioned before, it's important to look up and out as it helps to remember the vastness of the sky when your world has shrunk, and so this also makes both walking and nature incredibly important to hope and healing.

Another suggestion is to get them, at the end of the day, to think of three things they're grateful for. Depending on where they are in their grief, this may be a challenge, but it can range from something really small like 'I'm grateful for my nice warm bed' to something more profound such as 'I'm grateful to my loved one for being part of my life, for all I learned from them and for their love'. Although it may require great effort during grief, shifting perspective in this way has been shown to improve wellbeing. However, proceed with sensitivity and caution with this for obvious reasons, particularly

with difficult losses, as some people may not feel ready to feel gratitude for anything after a traumatic experience and may resent any
perceived implication that they should.

Support groups and social media

It's perhaps just human nature for us to seek out our own tribe, and
this is certainly true in grief. It's likely the friends of your bereaved
client will not be experiencing what they are currently going through,
so it can be helpful to seek solace by finding people who are. The two
main ways of doing this are support groups and via social media.

Support groups can be especially important for bereaved parents
and those who have lost a partner. They can provide comfort by
connecting you with people who share your experience when those
around you are unlikely to fully understand. Support groups can ward
off loneliness and isolation and they can also provide role models.
Seeing someone who has experienced a similar loss but is further
down the line – and surviving – can provide a sense of what the future
might be like and that it is, indeed, survivable. They can share advice
on dealing with Christmas and other festivals, anniversaries or other
people's lack of understanding and compassion. This advice is likely
to be more pertinent than any given by someone who hasn't 'lived
experience'. Groups also allow everyone's voice to be heard and their
individual grief to be witnessed within the collective, and this can
be such an important part of the grieving process. There are support
groups listed in the Appendix so that you're able to signpost your client
to the appropriate group. As is often said to newly bereaved parents
attending their first group meeting of The Compassionate Friends:
'Welcome to the group that no one wants to belong to.'

For many bereaved people, social media provides both a community and an avenue to vent and express their misery. The guidance
on this that I would suggest you pass on to your client is to proceed
with caution. I speak in *Love Untethered* about how, when I was first

bereaved, much of my current social media feeds felt completely irrelevant to me:

> Generally speaking, my advice is to cull everything on social media that is no longer in tune with your new existence and follow people and pages that resonate in the present moment. You may be drawn to closed Facebook groups for the bereaved, as I was, but if you find they are pulling you down, you may want to look for more balanced alternatives. As a bereaved person, you're already in pain – but you don't need to actively feed that pain, so look for those groups that acknowledge the reality of a tragic bereavement but that also demonstrate a hope that grief can at least soften, that your bond continues and, if appropriate to you, a belief that all life continues, just in a different form.[15]

Don't actively feed the pain would be my key takeaway here, as this could be a pitfall that could be very easy for your client to fall into regarding social media. About a year into bereavement, I set up an Instagram account[16] to post almost solely about grief in what I perceive to be a balanced way. I try to tread the line between acknowledging the undeniable pain of a significant loss and offering hope that it is possible to survive by continuing your bond with them. I find the grief community on Instagram to be really supportive, and several grief coaching clients have come to me via this platform. Creating posts to support others who are grieving has really helped me, and from what I can see, it seems to help others doing the same – perhaps it might help your client, too.

Books

Reading was what I turned to first when I lost my son. Many bereaved people seem unable to read initially (brain fog, lack of concentration,

---

15   May, 2022, p.157
16   @may.wellbeing

etc.), but I felt an overwhelming need to learn about grief, how other people in my position experienced it and what happens after death, in order to make some sense of what had happened to me. I have now read a huge number of books on grief, trauma and life after death – some are better than others, but they all offered me something of value. Whether I'm working with a client through nutritional therapy, wellbeing coaching or grief coaching, I quite often like to offer some reading material. If a grieving client doesn't feel up to reading at first, they perhaps will later on, so here are some recommendations that you may like to pass on. I also offer a little explanation for each so you can judge which one might be appropriate for the individual circumstances and needs of each client. I also share some films on grief which may be preferable for those who aren't big readers, as well as some podcasts.

Finding Meaning: The Sixth Stage of Grief, David Kessler (Rider, 2019)

David Kessler has been referred to on several occasions throughout this book and is considered a leading expert in the field of grief. This book covers the loss of his son, although it is by no means just aimed at readers who have lost a child. In fact, the main focus of the book is on post-traumatic growth and how important it can be to find a purpose and meaning in your life again after a loss. However, at the same time, he fully acknowledges that some losses can have a life-long impact. This is probably the book I recommend most often to my clients who are bereaved. David Kessler aims to offer a road map for grief, assisting the reader in eventually remembering those who have died with more love than pain.

Man's Search for Meaning, Viktor E. Frankl (Rider, 2004)

This is such an inspirational book and could be recommended for anyone really, whether they're grieving or not. It charts Frankl's life amid the horrors of the Nazi death camps and how this led to the formulation of his theory of logotherapy, based his own experience, which is an approach that can enable a person to transcend suffering and find a meaning to life, regardless of what has happened to them. The book is applicable to those who are grieving, because he demonstrates that even in the worst, most unendurable and seemingly impossible situation, we have the freedom to choose our attitude to it. 'When we are no longer able to change a situation, we are challenged to change ourselves.'

The Year of Magical Thinking, Joan Didion (Harper Perennial, 2006), and *Blue Nights*, Joan Didion (Fourth Estate, 2012)
These are beautifully written books about Joan Didion's experience of the loss of both her husband and her daughter. There is a certain detachment in her writing style, and her descriptions can at times appear stark, but there is an honesty to the shocking contrast between her seemingly glamourous life before her losses and her life afterwards. The way she writes is very compelling.

Resilient Grieving: Finding Strength and Embracing Life after a Loss That Changes Everything, Lucy Hone (The Experiment, 2017)
Lucy Hone is a psychologist from New Zealand who is also a bereaved mother. Her book is primarily about developing resilience. It's an excellent book, with lots of practical advice, and I've included it because it inspires hope for living a good, albeit different, life after a tragic loss. She does, however, appear to perhaps cope better than most bereaved parents I've so far come across. Nevertheless, if you have a client who currently feels hopeless about the future, this might be a good choice.

It's OK That You're Not OK: Meeting Grief and Loss in a Culture That Doesn't Understand, Megan Devine (Sounds True, 2017), and *How to Carry What Can't Be Fixed: A Journal for Grief*, Megan Devine (Sounds True, 2020)
It's OK That You're Not OK is another of my go-to recommendations for grieving clients, and it was, in fact, the first grief book I read. Devine begins it by writing: 'Here's what I most want to you to know: this really is as bad as you think.' (p. 3). She is brutally honest and very

angry that our culture treats grief as if it's a disease that needs to be somehow cured as quickly as possible. She rejects the 'five stages of grief' model as damaging and abhors that the bereaved have to suffer the pain of being judged, dismissed and misunderstood on top of their actual grief. As both a therapist and as a woman who witnessed the accidental drowning of her partner, she believes in building a life alongside grief rather than seeking to overcome it, and offers realistic advice on how you might do this. I love this book.

Devine's second book, *How to Carry What Can't Be Fixed*, is full of self-care exercises, practical advice and writing prompts to use during the grieving process. It's an attractively illustrated workbook which may appeal to some of your clients.

Permission to Mourn, Tom Zuba (Bish Press, 2014), and *Becoming Radiant*, Tom Zuba (Bish Press, 2018)

In contrast to the matter-of-fact tone of *It's OK That You're Not OK*, this is lovely, uplifting hopeful prose from a man who has experienced the deaths of two children and his wife. He offers 'a new way to do grief'. Because of the way they're written, they are great books to dip into – so a good recommendation for someone with brain fog or who is unable to concentrate. There's also a sense of if he can survive so many losses, then maybe you can, too. 'Grief is not the enemy. Grief can be one of our greatest teachers.' (p. 54).

What the Dead Are Dying to Teach Us, Claire Broad (Watkins Publishing, 2019)

This would only be appropriate for someone who has an interest in life after death. Claire is a medium, and I've had three readings with her that were all amazingly accurate. She is down to earth, and the book is well researched as Claire highlights findings from consciousness studies that she uses to challenge our understanding of the world. She discusses what we can learn from those already on the other side in order to make the most of this life while we are here – which is going to be comforting for a bereaved client with a spiritual interest.

Signs: The Secret Language of the Universe,
Laura Lynne Jackson (Piatkus, 2019)

This is another recommendation for any client who is interested in developing their spiritual connection. Considered a 'modern guide' to connecting with the other side, this book is how to recognize and interpret messages from loved ones. Laura Lynne Jackson helps to demystify this subject and provide an understanding that 'the secret language of the universe' is something available to everyone, not just mediums or psychics. It's inspiring and motivational yet also practical. Although there are many books written about the afterlife, this one and Claire Broad's book are my favourites.

I have already referred to my own book, *Love Untethered: How to Live When Your Child Dies* (Ayni Books, 2022), so all I will say here is that if you encounter a bereaved parent or anyone who has experienced another type of traumatic loss, I hope it might be of interest or of help.

Recommended films about grief

- *Rabbit Hole* (Nicole Kidman, Aaron Eckhart, Dianne Wiest), 2010.
- *Collateral Beauty* (Will Smith, Edward Norton, Keira Knightly), 2016.
- *Manchester by the Sea* (Casey Affleck, Michelle Williams), 2016.
- *Ordinary People* (Donald Sutherland, Mary Tyler Moore, Timothy Hutton), 1980.
- *Three Colours: Blue* (Juliette Binoche), 1993.

Podcasts for grief

- *Shapes of Grief* – a podcast by Liz Gleeson, bereavement therapist.
- *Griefcast* – a podcast hosted by comedian Cariad Lloyd.

Crystals

My list of suggestions you could make to your grieving client could go on and on, but one final mention is going to crystals. They may not take away the pain of grief, and their benefits have not been proven by science, but, in my experience, they can soothe the soul a little and this is what we're aiming for here. It's great that crystals are growing in popularity at the moment. Different crystals have different properties, and holding crystals or placing them on your body is thought to promote physical, emotional and spiritual healing by positively interacting with your body's energy field. I think when you are suffering from trauma and grief, simply holding something solid and beautiful can be a comfort in itself, and therefore this makes them worthy of suggestion to some grieving clients.

Crystals that are thought to be particularly beneficial for grief include black obsidian, lepidolite, apache tear, amethyst, rose quartz, smoky quartz.

Getting your client to fill their self-care basket with any of the above – and anything in addition they might like to add – is one way you can aid them in easing their path through grief, alongside your own professional expertise. These ideas may help them to see that healing is possible, that doing anything that brings peace and/or connection can counter some of their sorrow, and that it *is* possible to feel a little joy alongside it. If the loss was a major one, then they will need to fully comprehend that there is no going back to how they were pre-loss. They will have to find a way to go forward somehow, and I hope that some of these tools may assist in this. *However*, please be aware that, depending on the loss, this is a work in progress and one that may, in some cases, be a lifetime's work. In addition, helping them to set small achievable goals and encouraging them to say no to anything that they don't want to do are other ways you can support and empower them through their grief.

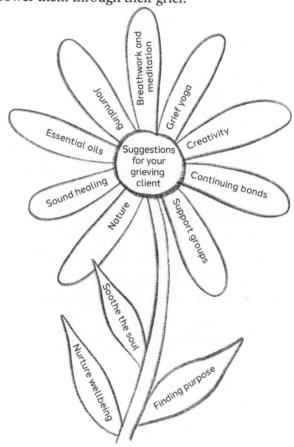

Suggestions for practical tools to use when coping with anxiety felt during grief

A simple exercise for your client to help them to calm down and redirect their thoughts into the present moment is to take notice of:

- five things you can see

- four things you can touch
- three things you can hear
- two things you can smell
- one emotion you feel.

Other techniques that can help create space away from the upsetting feelings experienced with anxiety or PTSD in grief include the following:

- Put your hands in water, going from hot to cold and focusing on the difference in how they feel.
- Pick something up (a crystal would be good here). How does it feel? Rough or smooth? What colour is it?
- Finger breathing technique: slowly inhale as you trace up one side of your finger, and exhale as you trace down the other side.
- Walk and count your steps and focus on their rhythm – putting one foot in front of another takes you forward literally and metaphorically.
- Choose a mantra such as 'I am safe, this is now'.
- Shaking out hands and feet can energetically release stagnant energy.
- Stamp your feet – this is apparently good for the adrenal glands, which are responsible for producing stress hormones.
- Visualize putting your grief and trauma in a box and putting it on a high shelf. You're not denying it's there, but you're just giving yourself a temporary break from it when you feel especially overwhelmed.
- Touch something comforting, a blanket, a smooth stone or a warm mug.
- Think of five things that give you joy – these may need to be very simple during grief, such as the sun on your face, chocolate, a TV programme.

I hope that this final chapter has provided you with some tools, resources and ideas to use or share with your grieving client, whatever type of grief they are experiencing, whether their loss is one which they will be able to assimilate into their life relatively soon or one that has left them profoundly changed.

Cheryl Strayed summarizes this beautifully:

> It's your life. The one you must make in the obliterated place that's now your world, where everything you used to be is simultaneously erased and omnipresent... The obliterated place is equal parts destruction and creation. The obliterated place is pitch black and bright light. It is water and parched earth. It is mud and it is manna. The real work of grief is making a home there.[17]

---

17   Strayed, 2013, p.282

Afterword

I hope that having read this book, you now stand better equipped to work confidently with a grieving client and that you feel you have an increased understanding of the complexity of grief – from the natural order of losing a parent or grandparent in old age to the tragedy of losing a baby or child; from learning about secondary losses to how grief can affect our mind, body and spirit. I hope if you had any fear or dread of working with a grieving client, this has now lessened and that you feel you have enough knowledge, tools and resources to support your client on what is likely, to a greater or lesser degree, to be a challenging path for them.

SELF-CARE AND BOUNDARIES

It may be that you're drawn to the work you do because you consider yourself to be an empath. There is no doubt that it can be especially heartbreaking to witness someone's deep grief, so to be a healthy empath you definitely need to have strong boundaries in place. This is also very important for your client. If they see you taking on their pain, they might feel that you'll be unable to support them in the way that they need. If we go into feeling their pain, we will lose not only our boundaries but theirs, too. So rather than focusing on the need to have empathy for someone who is grieving, it's perhaps more helpful to focus on compassion. Empathetic people feel the suffering of the person in pain, whereas compassionate people feel loving kindness towards them, which is healthier for both of you. Taking on their pain serves neither you nor your grieving client. Always try to leave their grief with them at the end of the session.

Contrary to what you might imagine about any extra demands of working with bereaved people, my experience has been that they are the least demanding of all of my clients in many ways, and very respectful of my boundaries. They are actually rather 'low maintenance', and it's probably pretty unlikely that they will bother you with tearful phone calls or distressed emails. In fact, ironically, you may find your clients who have comparatively far less to deal with contact you a great deal more and place far more demands on your time and energy than a grieving client. With boundaries firmly established, I will often send through an email between appointments with a link I've seen that might be of interest to them or a simple 'thinking of you' when I know they have a loved one's birthday or anniversary to get through. These small gestures always seem to be greatly appreciated and cost little of our time.

I am often asked whether working with others who are grieving is triggering for my own grief, especially when working with other bereaved mothers or widows, but that's not usually the case. I feel great compassion for my bereaved clients, but I seem able to draw a line after each session. Even if I think of them between appointments, it doesn't adversely affect my own equilibrium – maybe that's because I'm experienced at establishing boundaries or maybe it's because having my own great losses to bear, I have a natural protective mechanism and simply no additional room to embody the pain of others. And this means I am more able to support them effectively.

However, as a nutritional therapist, I learned early on that when I felt drained by certain clients, I could envisage a protective bubble around me so my energy remained mine. I also used a clearing aromatherapy spray after they had left. I think working online, as many of us do these days, offers a certain protection via the screen and from not being physically close to someone else's energy. A short meditation or affirmation before and after your client might also help if that's something you're inclined to do. But I really don't think bereaved clients will drain your energy more than any other client might. I also believe if you're not striving to fix the unfixable and you have built trust and rapport, then this won't be an issue. I don't view grieving clients as emotionally challenging to work with and therefore they don't seem to be.

Unless you specialize in grief as I do, then it's unlikely you'll be dealing with grieving clients too frequently, and when you do, not all of them will have suffered a traumatic loss or be in very early grief. If you really feel out of your depth (which I hope won't now be the case!), then refer on for both your sake and the sake of the client. And you will, of course, always refer on if you feel there is a serious physical or mental health issue or suicide risk.

A couple of additional small points you might like to consider.

One is becoming a trauma-informed practitioner. There is currently more awareness for trauma than there is for grief, although unfortunately that increased awareness has led to a certain trivialization – people will say 'I'm traumatized' or 'I think I've got PTSD' about anything they feel to be vaguely upsetting, diminishing the true horror of trauma. However, I feel being a trauma-informed or trauma-aware practitioner will become more common and perhaps, one day, even be a requirement. There are lots of CPD-type course available online if you want to pursue this. This would then enable you to feel confident in dealing not only with clients who have experienced a traumatic loss, but with those who have been through other types of traumas, too.

You might also like to add a question specifically about bereavements to your questionnaire if you use one, asking about the relationship (mother, friend, brother, etc.), the date of the loss, and possibly whether the client still feels affected by the loss, and if so, how. This will mean you will feel prepared, can refer to the relevant chapters in this book in advance and be able to start to make any potential links between the bereavement and their symptoms.

Why you are needed

We need to become a more grief-literate society so that we stop being so terrified of death and of the bereaved. We are all likely to experience loss at some point in our lives and we are all going to die. This really shouldn't be a taboo subject because that just reinforces the fear. As you will now be aware, those who have lost a child or have had a loved one die by suicide, overdose or murder report feeling stigmatized, as if what's happened to them is in some way contagious. This is simply not right. If you, as a grief-aware practitioner, can hold space for these clients and are unafraid to witness their pain and trauma having read the guidance in this book, then you will be offering a truly valuable service. The more grief-aware we are as practitioners and as a society, the more resilient grieving people can become.

Appendix

KEY ORGANIZATIONS

You may find the following a useful list to refer your client to. It's primarily a UK-based list, although I have listed some organizations outside the UK. If you are outside the UK, you should be able to find an equivalent organization to those listed below.

Cruse Bereavement Support

Cruse is the UK's largest bereavement charity, providing advice and information on support groups and bereavement counselling to people suffering from grief of all kinds. They have a free helpline.

www.cruse.org.uk

The Good Grief Trust

An alternative umbrella organization to Cruse that is rapidly growing, again covering all types of grief. The Good Grief Guide is run by the bereaved, for the bereaved. They're very active on social media and say they aim to be the UK's leading fully comprehensive online bereavement service, bringing bereavement into the 21st century and changing the perception we have of grief in this country.

www.thegoodgrieftrust.org

The Compassionate Friends

The Compassionate Friends website is specifically for families who have lost a child of any age. They provide an incredible range of information, everything from advice on inquests to loss through murder or suicide, plus retreats and a helpline run by bereaved parents. Their individual sections are enormously helpful – there's nothing they haven't covered.

www.tcf.org.uk

For siblings: www.tcf.org.uk/content/ftb-siblings

For grandparents: www.tcf.org.uk/content/ftb-grandparents

Outside the UK:

US: www.compassionatefriends.org

Canada: http://tcfcanada.net

Australia: https://tcfa.org.au

WAY

WAY stands for widowed and young, and is a charity based in the UK, offering peer-to-peer support, understanding and friendship for anyone who has lost a partner before their 51st birthday – married or not, with or without children, inclusive of sexual orientation, gender, race and religion.

www.widowedandyoung.org.uk

Soaring Spirits International

Soaring Spirits builds a community through grief support programmes for widowed men and women, serving a worldwide population, and endeavouring to ensure no one grieves alone. Soaring Spirits is an inclusive, non-denominational organization focused on hope and healing through the grieving process, offering members the tools and resources they need to rebuild their lives in the aftermath of the death of a spouse or life partner.

https://soaringspirits.org

The Dinner Party

The Dinner Party is a platform for grieving 20–30-somethings to find peer community. The Dinner Party mission is to transform the difficult conversations around grief into candid conversation and forward movement using the age-old practice of gathering and breaking bread. The idea is you join a virtual table. Dinner party times are US-based but open to anyone wherever in the world they might live.

www.thedinnerparty.org

The Coroners' Court Support Service

The Coroners' Court Support Service provide volunteers who will come with you to an inquest, talk you through the process on the day and just generally provide kindness and support. There is also a helpline and lots of links to information on their website to help you understand the inquest process, which can be so very daunting:

https://coronerscourtssupportservice.org.uk

They also have a page that has useful links to organizations that specialize in various types of unexpected death, such as drugs or alcohol, road accidents, stillbirths, etc.

https://coronerscourtssupportservice.org.uk/useful-links-organisations

Sudden

This organization provides information specifically on coping with a sudden bereavement, whether due to accident, sudden event or suicide. They provide online help and guidance with links to more specific help, depending on how the person died.

www.sudden.org/help-for-adults

At a Loss

A signposting website, directing the bereaved to the most appropriate services. There is a section specifically for 18–30-year-olds who have been bereaved and a section for men (who sometimes don't seek support or talk through their grief in the way women do). There is also a counsellor live chat service.

www.ataloss.org

If you are concerned that your client is suicidal

As previously mentioned, suicidal ideation is not unusual if someone has experienced a traumatic loss, and you may want to provide your client with the following information.

The Samaritans

www.samaritans.org

Call: 116 123

StayAlive

The StayAlive app is a suicide prevention resource for the UK. Useful information and tools to help those at risk of suicide and people worried about them.

www.stayalive.app

The Campaign Against Living Miserably (CALM)
CALM, a leading movement against suicide, run a free, confidential and anonymous helpline as well as a web chat service, offering help, advice and information to anyone who is struggling or in crisis.

www.thecalmzone.net

Call: 0800 585858

References

Albom, M. (2009). *Tuesdays with Morrie: An Old Man, a Young Man, and Life's Greatest Lesson*. Sphere.

Aoun, S.M., Breen, L.J., Rumbold, B., Christian, K.M., Same, A. and Abel, J. (2019). 'Matching response to need: What makes social networks fit for providing bereavement support?' *PLoS ONE,* 14(3), e0213367. doi.org/10.1371/journal.pone.0213367 2019

APA (2022). *Diagnostic and Statistical Manual of Mental Disorders*, 5th edition, Text Revision (DSM-5-TR™). American Psychiatric Association.

Baikie, K.A. and Wilhelm, K. (2005). 'Emotional and physical health benefits of expressive writing'. *Advances in Psychiatric Treatment,* 11(5), 338–346. doi.org/10.1192/apt.11.5.338

Bakalar, N. (2021). 'The loss of a child takes a physical toll on the heart'. *New York Times.* www.nytimes.com/2021/11/23/well/family/death-of-a-child-parents-heart-attack-risk.html.

BetterSleep (n.d.). 'The science behind Solfeggio frequencies'. www.better-sleep.com/blog/science-behind-solfeggio-frequencies.

Bowlby, J. (1997). *Attachment and Loss Trilogy*. Pimlico.

Brown, B. (2020). 'PTSD: Building resilience to trauma-induced mental health issues with a functional medicine approach'. *IHCAN.* www.ihcan-mag.com/imag/ihcanjuly20/index.html

Cacciatore, J. (2017). *Bearing the Unbearable: Love, Loss, and the Heartbreaking Path of Grief*. Wisdom Publications.

Calaprice, A. (ed.) (2002). *Dear Professor Einstein: Albert Einstein's Letters to and from Children*. Prometheus Books.

Cankaya, B., Chapman, B.P., Talbot, N.L, Moynihan, J., and Duberstein, P.R. (2009). 'History of sudden unexpected loss is associated with elevated interleukin-6 and decreased insulin-like growth factor-1 in women in an urban primary care setting'. *Psychosomatic Medicine, 71*(9), 914–919. doi.org/10.1097/psy.0b013e3181be7aa8

Chandrasekhar, K., Kapoor, J. and Anishetty, S. (2012). 'A prospective, randomized double-blind, placebo-controlled study of safety and efficacy of a high-concentration full-spectrum extract of ashwagandha root in reducing stress and anxiety in adults'. *Indian Journal of Psychological Medicine, 34*(3), 255–262. doi:10.4103/0253-7176.106022

Cheung, T. and Broad, C. (2017). *Answers from Heaven*. Piatkus.

Childs, E. and de Wit, H. (2014). 'Regular exercise is associated with emotional resilience to acute stress in healthy adults'. *Frontiers in Physiology, 5*, 161. doi:10.3389/fphys.2014.00161

Christopherson, B., (n.d.). 'The Elephant in the room of grief'. *Social Work Today*. www.socialworktoday.com/archive/exc_0316.shtml

Church, D. and Feinstein, D. (2007). 'The manual stimulation of acupuncture points in the treatment of post-traumatic stress disorder: A review of clinical emotional freedom techniques'. *Medical Acupuncture, 29*(4), 194–205. doi:10.1089/acu.2017.1213

Cox, C.J., Cooper, C.E. and Smith, M.D. (2017). 'Exploring the effects of mediumship on hope, resilience, and post-traumatic growth in the bereaved'. *Journal of Exceptional Experiences and Psychology, 5*(2), 6–15.

Delagran, L. (n.d.). 'How does nature impact our wellbeing?' Earl E. Bakken Center for Spirituality and Healing, University of Minnesota. www.takingcharge.csh.umn.edu/how-does-nature-impact-our-wellbeing

Devine, M. (2014). 'If it isn't meant to "cure" grief, what good is therapy?' HuffPost. www.huffpost.com/entry/grief-therapy_b_5077196

Devine, M. (2017). *It's OK That You're Not OK: Meeting Grief and Loss in a Culture That Doesn't Understand*. Sounds True.

Ding, N., Li, L., Song, K., Huang, A. and Zhang, A. (2020). 'Efficacy and safety of acupuncture in treating post-traumatic stress disorder: A protocol for systematic review and meta-analysis'. *Medicine (Baltimore), 99*(26), e20700. doi:10.1097/MD.0000000000020700

Dmitrašinović, G., Pešić, V., Stanić, D., *et al.* (2016). 'ACTH, cortisol and IL-6 levels in athletes following magnesium supplementation'. *Journal of Medical Biochemistry, 35*(4), 375–384. doi:10.1515/jomb-2016-0021

Dwyer, W. (1989). *You'll See It When You Believe It: The Way to Your Personal Transformation*. Random House.

Fagundes, C.P., Brown, R.L, Chen, M.A., Murdock, K.W., *et al.* (2019). 'Grief, depressive symptoms, and inflammation in the spousally bereaved'. *Psychoneuroendocrinology, 100*, 190–197. doi.org/10.1016/j.psyneuen.2018.10.006

Fossella, T. (2011). 'Human nature, Buddha nature: An interview with John Welwood'. *Tricycle: The Buddhist Review*. https://tricycle.org/magazine/human-nature-buddha-nature

Frogge, S. (2015). 'The myth of divorce following the death of a child'. TAPS. www.taps.org/articles/21-1/divorce

Gann, C. (2011). 'Grieving parents face higher risk of early death, study says'. *ABC News*. https://abcnews.go.com/Health/grieving-parents-risk-early-death-study/story?id=14467734

Gesser, G., Wong, P.T.P. and Reker, G.T. (1988). ' Death attitudes across the life span: The development and validation of the Death Attitude Profile (DAP)'. *Omega*, 2, 113–128. doi.org/10.2190%2F0DQB-7Q1E-2BER-H6YC

Gibson-Smith, D., Bot, M., Brouwer, I.A., Visser, M., and Penninx, B.W.J.H. (2018). 'Diet quality in persons with and without depressive and anxiety disorders'. *Journal of Psychiatric Research*, 106, 1–7. doi.org/10.1016/j.jpsychires.2018.09.006

Gray, T. (2016). 'Your health and grief'. Psych Central. https://psychcentral.com/lib/your-health-and-grief#1. Accessed 2021.

Greenblatt, J. (2016). 'Magnesium: The missing link in mental health?' Integrative Medicine for Mental Health. www.greatplainslaboratory.com/articles-1/2016/11/17/magnesium-the-missing-link-in-mental-health

Harris, N. (2014). '4 reasons journaling is good for you'. *Good Housekeeping*. https://www.goodhousekeeping.com/health/wellness/advice/a25762/health-benefits-journaling

Havening Techniques (n.d.). 'FAQs: The Havening Techniques FAQs'. www.havening.org/about-havening/faqs

Hayes, A. (2020). 'Bob Geldof still breaks down weeping over "clever, sweet, eccentric" Peaches'. *Sky News*. https://news.sky.com/story/bob-geldof-still-breaks-down-weeping-over-clever-sweet-eccentric-peaches-11947154

Heslop, J. [Manifest by Jess] (2019, Aug 19). 10 minute Chakra Meditation (Daily Recharge) [Video]. YouTube. www.youtube.com/watch?v=o89px3RWFS8

Hyman, Dr M. (Host). (2019, Feb 20). 'Why Meditation is the New Medicine' (No. 41) [Audio podcast episode]. In The Doctor's Farmacy with Mark Hyman, M.D. https://drhyman.com/blog/2019/02/20/podcast-ep41

Kar, N. (2011). 'Cognitive behavioral therapy for the treatment of post-traumatic stress disorder: A review'. *Neuropsychiatric Disease and Treatment*, 7, 167–181. doi:10.2147/NDT.S10389

Kessler, D. (n.d.) Grief.com: Because love never dies. https://grief.com

Kessler, D. (2019). *Finding Meaning: The Sixth Stage of Grief.* Rider.

Kim, S., Jo, K., Hong, K.-B., Han, S.H. and Suh, H.J. (2019). 'GABA and l-theanine mixture decreases sleep latency and improves NREM sleep'. *Pharmaceutical Biology*, 57(1), 65–73. doi:10.1080/13880209.2018.1557698

King, K. (2020). 'Grief and loss: Will therapists be able to help? The next pandemic will be one of grief – and many therapists are not ready'. *Psychology Today*. www.psychologytoday.com/us/blog/lifespan-perspectives/202008/grief-and-loss-will-therapists-be-able-help

Klass, D., Silverman, P.R. and Nickman, S. (1996). *Continuing Bonds: New Understandings of Grief*. Routledge.

Knowles, L.M., Ruiz, J.M., and O'Connor, M.-F. (2019). 'A systematic review of the association between bereavement and biomarkers of immune function'. *Psychosomatic Medicine*, 81(5), 415–433. doi:10.1097/PSY.0000000000000693

Kübler-Ross, E. (2014). *On Death and Dying: What the Dying Have to Teach Doctors, Nurses, Clergy and Their Own Families*, 50th anniversary edition. Scribner.

Levine, P. (n.d.) www.somaticexperiencing.com

Lewis, C.S. (2013). *A Grief Observed*. Faber & Faber.

Li, B., Lv, J., Wang, W. and Zhang, D. (2016). 'Dietary magnesium and calcium intake and risk of depression in the general population: A meta-analysis'. *Australian and New Zealand Journal of Psychiatry*, 51(3), 219–229. doi.org/10.1177/0004867416676895

Lipinski, K. (2012). 'Reiki and post-traumatic stress disorder'. The International Center for Reiki Training. www.reiki.org/articles/reiki-and-post-traumatic-stress-disorder

Lopresti, A.L. and Drummond, P.D. (2014). 'Saffron (Crocus sativus) for depression: A systematic review of clinical studies and examination of underlying antidepressant mechanisms of action'. *Human Psychopharmacology*, 29(6), 517–527. doi:10.1002/hup.2434

Lynch, P. (n.d.). 'EFT "tapping" for PTSD'. PTSD UK. www.ptsduk.org/eft-tapping-for-ptsd/8

May, V. (2022). *Love Untethered: How to Live When Your Child Dies*. Ayni Books.

Moody, R.A. (1993). *Reunions: Visionary Encounters with Departed Loved Ones*. Villard Books.

Moritz, B., Schmitz, A.E., Rodrigues, A.L.S., Dafre, A.L. and Cunha, M.P. (2020). 'The role of vitamin C in stress-related disorders'. *Journal of Nutritional Biochemistry*, 85, 108459. doi:10.1016/j.jnutbio.2020.108459

Navarro, P.N., Landin-Romero, R., Guardiola-Wanden-Berghe, R., Moreno-Alcázar, A., *et al.* (2018). '25 years of Eye Movement Desensitization and Reprocessing (EMDR): The EMDR therapy protocol, hypotheses of its mechanism of action and a systematic review of its efficacy in the treatment of post-traumatic stress disorder'. *Revista de Psiquiatría y Salud Mental*, 11(2), 101–114 (English edition). doi:10.1016/j.rpsm.2015.12.002

NICE (2018a). 'Emotional freedom techniques: What is the clinical and cost effectiveness of emotional freedom techniques (EFT) for the treatment of PTSD in adults?' National Institute for Health and Care Excellence. www.nice.org.uk/researchrecommendation/what-is-the-clinical-and-cost-effectiveness-of-emotional-freedom-techniques-eft-for-the-treatment-of-ptsd-in-adults

NICE (2018b). *Post-traumatic Stress Disorder*. NICE guideline NG116. https://www.nice.org.uk/guidance/ng116/evidence/d-psychological-psychosocial-and-other-nonpharmacological-interventions-for-the-treatment-of-ptsd-in-adults-pdf-6602621008

Nussinovitch, U., Goitein, O., Nussinovitch, N., and Altman, A. (2011). 'Distinguishing a heart attack from the "broken heart syndrome" (Takotsubo cardiomyopathy)'. *Journal of Cardiovascular Nursing*, 26(6), 524–529. doi:10.1097/JCN.0b013e31820e2a90

O'Mahony, S.M., Clarke, G., Borre, Y.E., Dinan, T.G., and Cryan, J.F. (2015). 'Serotonin, tryptophan metabolism and the brain-gut-microbiome axis'. *Behavioural Brain Research*, 277. doi:10.1016/j.bbr.2014.07.027.6

Pedersen, T. (2022). 'Your health and grief'. Psych Central. https://psychcentral.com/lib/your-health-and-grief

Pitman, A., Rantell, K., Marston, L., King, M. and Osborn, D. (2017). 'Perceived stigma of sudden bereavement as a risk factor for suicidal thoughts and suicide attempt: Analysis of British cross-sectional survey data on 3387 young bereaved adults'. *International Journal of Environmental Research and Public Health*, 14(3), 286. doi.org/10.3390/ijerph14030286

Pitstick, M.R. (2006). *Soul Proof*. Soul Proof Productions.

PTSD UK (n.d.(a)). 'Causes of post traumatic stress disorder'. www.ptsduk.org/what-is-ptsd/causes-of-ptsd

PTSD UK (n.d.(b)). 'Cognitive behavioural therapy (CBT)'. www.ptsduk.org/treatment-help/cognitive-behavioural-therapy-cbt

Renehan, E.J. Jr. (2002). *The Kennedys at War*. Knopf Doubleday.

Sagan, C. (2008). *The Demon-Haunted World: Science as a Candle in the Dark*, reprint edition. Paw Prints.

Savonix (2018). 'Magnesium: The one supplement this neuroscientist CEO takes every day'. https://savonix.com/blog/one-supplement-neuroscientist-ceo-takes-every-day

Scentered (2020). 'How essential oils affect your limbic system'. https://scentered.me/blogs/news/how-essential-oils-affect-your-limbic-system

Schutten, J.C., Joris, P.J., Minović, I., *et al.* (2021). 'Long-term magnesium supplementation improves glucocorticoid metabolism: A post-hoc analysis of an intervention trial'. *Clinical Endocrinology*, 94(2), 150–157. doi:10.1111/cen.14350

Seiler, A., von Känel, R. and Slavich, G.M. (2020). 'The psychobiology of bereavement and health: A conceptual review from the perspective of social signal transduction theory of depression'. *Frontiers in Psychiatry*, 11, 565239. doi:10.3389/fpsyt.2020.565239

Shapiro, F. (2014). 'The role of eye movement desensitization and reprocessing (EMDR) therapy in medicine: Addressing the psychological and physical symptoms stemming from adverse life experiences'. *Permanente Journal*, 18(1), 71–77. doi:10.7812/TPP/13-098

Shulman, L.M. (2018). 'Loss: A neurologist's perspective on loss, grief and the brain'. Johns Hopkins University Press. https://press.prod.jhu.mindgrb.io/newsroom/and-after-loss-neurologists-perspective-loss-grief-and-brain.

Strayed, C. (2013). *Tiny Beautiful Things*. Atlantic Books.

Tonkin, L. (1996). 'Growing around grief – another way of looking at grief and recovery'. *Bereavement Care*, 15(1). doi:10.1080/02682629608657376

Valentine, C., McKell, J. and Ford, A. (2017). 'Service failures and challenges in responding to people bereaved through drugs and alcohol: An inter-professional analysis'. *Journal of Interprofessional Care*, 32(3), 295–303. doi:10.1080/13561820.2017.1415312

Van Der Kolk, B. (2014). *The Body Keeps the Score: Brain, Mind, and Body in the Healing of Trauma*. Penguin.

Walsh, K., King, M., Jones, L., Tookman, A. and Blizard, R. (2002). 'Spiritual beliefs may affect outcome of bereavement: Prospective study'. *BMJ*, 324(7353), 1551. doi:10.1136/bmj.324.7353.1551

Wong, P. (2008). 'Transformation of grief through meaning: Meaning-centered counseling for bereavement'. www.drpaulwong.com/transformation-grief-meaning

Wong, P.T.P., Reker, G.T. and Gesser, G. (1994). 'Death Attitude Profile – Revised: A multidimensional measure of attitudes toward death (DAP-R)'. In R.A. Neimeyer (ed.) *Death Anxiety Handbook: Research, Instrumentation, and Application*. Taylor & Francis.

Worden, J.W. (2009). *Grief Counseling and Grief Therapy: A Handbook for the Mental Health Practitioner*, 4th edition. Routledge.

Young, L.M., Pipingas, A., White, D.J., Gauci, S. and Scholey, A. (2019). 'A systematic review and meta-analysis of B vitamin supplementation on depressive symptoms, anxiety, and stress: Effects on healthy and "at-risk" individuals'. *Nutrients*, 11(9), 2232. doi:10.3390/nu11092232

Zhai, Y. and Du, X. (2020). 'Loss and grief amidst COVID-19: A path to adaptation and resilience'. *Brain, Behavior, and Immunity*, 87, 80–81. doi. org/10.1016/j.bbi.2020.04.053

Zuba, T. (2018). *Becoming Radiant*. Bish Press.

About the Author

Vanessa May is a holistic grief coach, BANT nutritional therapist and ILM-accredited wellbeing coach from London. She has recently trained with leading grief expert David Kessler and is now a certified grief educator.

In her practice, Vanessa offers a unique type of bereavement support, looking at all aspects of the grieving process and how it can affect not only emotional and mental wellbeing but also the body and the spirit. She combines her lived experience of grief with her professional skill set to inform how she works with bereaved clients.

She wrote her first book, *Love Untethered*, in part to make sense of her profound grief and trauma, as well as in the hope that it can help others who have suffered a major loss.

She is now writing a third book which will explore grief beyond the first year, the impact of multiple losses and her personal experience of being both a bereaved mother and a widow.

Vanessa is passionate about improving our understanding of the diversity and complexity of grief and its potentially far-reaching effects on the mind, body and spirit.

- www.wellbeingandnutrition.co.uk
- www.vanessamay.co.uk (author website)
- Email: vanessa@wellbeingandnutrition.co.uk
- Instagram: @may.wellbeing
- Twitter: @maywellbeing